Male

Sexual Health

Male
Sexual Health

WRITTEN BY COLETTE PELLERIN

UNDER THE SUPERVISION OF Dr. MICHAEL McCORMACK

PREFACE BY GUY LAFLEUR

National Library of Canada cataloguing in publication

Main entry under title:

Male Sexual Health

Translation of: La santé sexuelle de l'homme.

ISBN 2-922260-10-0

1. Men - Health and hygiene. 2. Sexual disorders. 3. Impotence. 4. Generative organs, Male - Diseases. I. McCormack, Michael, 1953- .

RC875.S2613 2003   616.6'9   C2003-940749-7

Translation : Vera Roy

English editing : Anna Griffiths

Graphic design : Dino Peressini

Cover photo : François LeClair

Illustrations : Frank Renzo

© Rogers Media, 2003

1001 de Maisonneuve Blvd. West, 10th floor

Montreal (Quebec) H3A 3E1

Tel. : (514) 843-2542 ; fax : (514) 845-2063

E-mail : mhlivre@lactualite.com

Legal deposit : 2nd quarter 2003

Bibliothèque nationale du Québec, 2003

National Library of Canada, 2003

The publication of this work was made possible through an unrestricted educational grant from Pfizer Canada Inc.

Printed in Canada

COLLABORATORS :

Dr. Pierre Alarie

Family doctor and director of Sexual Dysfunction Unit,
Health Centre of the University of Montréal (CHUM)
Assistant Professor, Department of Family Medicine,
Faculty of Medicine, University of Montréal

Dr. François Bénard

Urologist and andrology specialist,
Health Centre of the University of Montréal (CHUM)
Associate clinical professor, Department of Surgery,
Faculty of Medicine, University of Montréal

Dr. Hélène Dugré

Family doctor and clinical psychologist, specialized in sexual medicine,
Sexual Dysfunction Unit, Health Centre of the University of Montréal (CHUM)
Clinical lecturer, Department of Family Medicine,
University of Montréal and University of Sherbrooke

Mr. Michel Goulet

Clinical sex therapist, Sexual Dysfunction Unit,
Health Centre of the University of Montréal (CHUM)
Professor, Department of Sexology, University of Québec at Montréal

Dr. Michael McCormack

Urologist, Health Centre of the University of Montréal (CHUM)
Associate professor, Department of Surgery,
Faculty of Medicine, University of Montréal

Dr. Luc Valiquette

Urologist, Health Centre of the University of Montréal (CHUM)
Professor, Department of Surgery,
Faculty of Medicine, University of Montréal

FROM THE SAME PUBLISHER

Dr. Jean-Louis Chiasson et al.
Understand your Diabetes... and Live a Healthy Life (2001)

Dr. André-H. Dandavino et al.
The Family Guide to Health Problems (2001)

Dr. Jacques Boulay
Bilingual Guide to Medical Abbreviations, 3rd edition (1998)

Table of contents

CHAPTER 3

OTHER TYPES OF SEXUAL DYSFUNCTION

Preface

When I was approached to speak publicly about male sexual dysfunction, at first I hesitated because the subject was still taboo. However, after discovering that one out of three Canadian men suffer from erectile dysfunction (ED), I decided that I would be glad to open the topic up for discussion and help men understand the importance of dealing with any of the sexual health problems they experience.

Over the last year, I have spoken to hundreds of men across the country who told me they did not regularly visit their doctors and only consulted a medical professional when they were very sick.

Few men can bring themselves to discuss sexual dysfunction openly with their doctor, which means that many cases remain undiagnosed. It also means that more serious health problems which may be at the root of the disorder remain undiagnosed as well.

For example, in cases of erectile dysfunction, statistics show that 75% of the time, this disorder is directly linked to another untreated medical condition, such as diabetes, prostate problems, or heart disease. However, since most men are reluctant to talk about the problem, only 15% of those with ED are diagnosed. Moreover, this reluctance means that it takes an average of three to five years for a man to actually consult a doctor after he has decided that he needs medical advice.

Men need to be proactive when it comes to sexual dysfunction and health in general. Yearly check-ups and open communication with a doctor are the keys to good health.

I am very proud to be helping others understand that sexual disorders are health problems, and that they should be discussed with a doctor. I hope this book will encourage more men to take control, and take better care of their health.

Guy Lafleur

Foreword

Men's sexual health is a timely subject. Over the last few years, particularly since sildenafil (better known as Viagra) proudly took its place on pharmacy shelves, people have been more openly addressing issues such as erectile dysfunction, premature ejaculation, performance anxiety and lowered sex drive. An incalculable number of television and radio programs, articles and Web sites have been devoted to various types of male sexual problems. Even though the amount of available information is growing, however, it is still quite rare to find a full-length work that touches on all the issues.

This book is an attempt to do just that. Based on interviews with experts, medical doctors and a sex therapist from the Health Center of the University of Montreal (CHUM), it provides an overview of the most common problems related to male sexuality in clear and accessible language. The goal of the book is to help the reader find pertinent information regarding the assessment, diagnosis and treatment of the most frequently encountered sexual disorders.

Who should I consult about erectile dysfunction – a family doctor, a specialist, or a sex therapist? What kind of examination should I undergo? Will the doctor prescribe Viagra? Is it a safe treatment? What are the alternative solutions? How can sex therapy help solve the problem of premature ejaculation? What can I do to get rid of performance anxiety? Is it normal to experience a decreased sex drive with the person I love ?

The following chapters will answer all these questions, and more. This book was written to help men – and couples – demystify male sexual dysfunction and find a satisfactory solution. By reading these words now, in fact, you are already on your way.

Dr. Serge Carrier
Urologist
Associate Professor of Surgery
McGill University

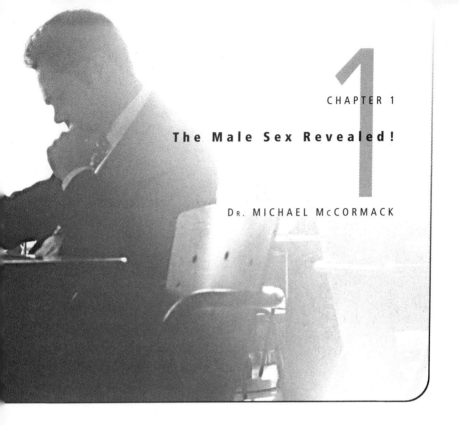

CHAPTER 1

The Male Sex Revealed!

D<small>R</small>. MICHAEL M<small>c</small>CORMACK

■ THE IMPORTANCE OF A SEX LIFE

For most people, making love is very important. More than simply a means of achieving physical pleasure, the sexual act is a powerful source of self-esteem. It makes a person feel attractive, gives them a sense of self-worth, and puts men and women alike fully in touch with their bodies. Sexuality, which can be expressed in various ways, is beneficial to a sense of personal balance.

In a couple, sex is the most intimate way a person has of saying "I love you" or "I want you" to his or her partner. Ideally, a couple's sexual relationship is an aspect of their communication – a way in which they express their harmony and shared happiness – and should therefore be an integral part of every couple's dynamic. Indeed, a couple's sexual relationship is often considered to be a barometer of the solidity of their relationship as a whole.

Not surprisingly, then, when a couple experiences some kind of sexual problem, a number of certainties can be called into question: doubts arise about self-image, how well the partners get along as a couple, the level of everyday personal satisfaction, to give only a few examples. This kind of self-questioning may be even more pronounced in men, for whom ideas of virility and performance are fundamental to defining their image in society. Furthermore, as well as worrying about his health, a man dealing with sexual dysfunction may also feel diminished and incapable, as though he were "not the man he used to be."

Statistics show that male sexual dysfunction is widespread. Fortunately, our knowledge of the subject has evolved a great deal since the 1980s, when it was thought that the majority of these problems were "all in the head." For example, because there was no clear understanding of the mechanics of erection, it was generally believed that most erectile dysfunction had a psychological cause. Doctors now know that in most cases physical health problems are responsible, and discoveries such as this have helped men come out of their shells and talk more openly about their sex lives.

Scientists continue to do research in the area of men's sexual health, since there is still so much to learn. And indeed, the issue is of increasing importance as the population grows older, life expectancies continue to rise, and most men and women expect to have sexual relations well into their golden years.

WHEN IN ROME...
The word testicle derives from the Latin *testis*, which means "witness." In Ancient Rome, men put their hands on their testicles in order to swear an oath, much like we place our hands on the Bible today.
The fact that women do not have testicles did not pose a problem for the Ancient Romans, since Roman women were not believed to have the capacity to swear oaths.

The sex life of elderly people has always been a bit of a taboo subject in our society. The appearance of sildenafil (Viagra), however, has made it much easier to talk about.

To learn more about the sexuality of people as they age, the pharmaceutical company Pfizer, Inc. undertook a massive study in 29 countries. They interviewed 26 000 people, both men and women, aged 40 to 80 (1000 Canadians took part in the study). The results were published in 2002.

The study showed that, among people in this age group:

- 83% of men and 63% of women say sex is important in their lives;
- 40% of women say that their partner's capacity does not diminish with age;
- 31% of men agree with this statement;
- 82% of men and 64% of women have had sexual relations in the last year (73% for both Canadian men and women);
- 57% of men and 51% of women made love from one to six times a week over the last year.

WHAT IS SPERM MADE OF?

Although the number of sperm in an average ejaculation can be anywhere from 20 to 100 million, this represents merely 1% of the total volume of the semen ejaculated. Substances produced by the prostate and seminal vesicles constitute the other 99%.

Some of these substances reduce the acidity of vaginal secretions so that sperm will not be destroyed. There are also amino acids and a large amount of fructose, a kind of sugar, which nourishes the sperm. Semen also contains prostaglandin. This chemical substance, when introduced into the vagina, produces muscle contractions in the woman that facilitate the movement of semen towards the uterus.

▨ ANATOMY OF THE MALE GENITALIA

The male genital and reproductive organs are men's primary sex characteristics. The most important are the testicles, the epididymis, the prostate, the seminal vesicles, the duct system and, of course, the penis.

The testicles are two oval-shaped organs that produce sperm. They are located below the abdomen and are enclosed in a pouch-like structure called the scrotum. Their position outside the body maintains the testicles at a temperature slightly lower (approximately 3 °C) than body temperature, which is essential to the production of viable sperm. As well as sperm, the testicles also manufacture 95% of the testosterone produced by the male body (the other 5% is produced by the adrenal glands). Testosterone is a hormone that plays an important role in the development and maintenance of male sexual function.

The epididymis are long, thin tubes located in the scrotum, along each testicle. Sperm are stored in the epididymis until ejaculation.

At the moment of ejaculation, the sperm leave the epididymes by the vas deferens. Along the way, they mix with the other components of semen that are secreted by the prostate and the seminal vesicles (*see frame, page 19, "What Is Sperm Made of?"*). The prostate is a gland

PENILE ANATOMY

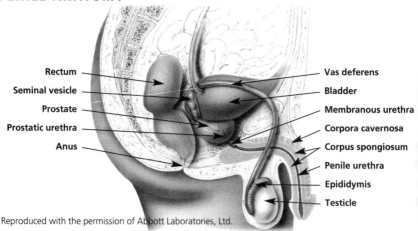

Rectum — Vas deferens
Seminal vesicle — Bladder
Prostate — Membranous urethra
Prostatic urethra — Corpora cavernosa
Anus — Corpus spongiosum
Penile urethra
Epididymis
Testicle

Reproduced with the permission of Abbott Laboratories, Ltd.

located below the bladder and is about the size of a golf ball. The seminal vesicles are little sac-like structures located on either side of the prostate. The semen then travels through the ejaculatory ducts and finally passes through the urethra to be discharged by the penis.

The penis (or phallus) is a structure of three parallel cylinders of spongy tissue. Two of the cylinders are called the corpora cavernosa (or cavernous bodies) and the third is known as the corpus spongiosum (or spongy body). Each consists of tissues which contain irregular cavities, like those in a sponge. At the end of the penis is the glans, which is approximately bell-shaped. At the very tip is the urethral orifice or meatus, through which urine and semen are expelled.

■ THE MARVELLOUS MECHANICS OF ERECTION

The mechanics of erection are highly complex. The following description will attempt as clear an explanation as possible. To begin, it is important to point out that although erection depends on a number of factors, voluntary control is not one of them. And, contrary to popular belief, not everything happens below the belt!

Erection is the result of a perfectly balanced process involving the brain, blood vessels, nerves and hormones, in particular testosterone.

When a man is sexually excited (through stimulation of the genital organs, fantasies or visual stimulation), the brain triggers a series of

IS THERE A BONE IN THE PENIS?
Yes, this does sound like a funny question!
However, it is interesting to note that in most mammals, there is indeed a bone in the penis. It is called the baculum, and its function is to make the penis erect. Humans, whales and ungulates (i.e., hoofed animals) are the only exceptions.

reactions which cause the nerves in the penis to release neurotransmitters, which in turn causes a dilation of the penile blood vessels. This dilation allows the penis to fill with blood. As the cavernous and spongy bodies become engorged, the veins that normally drain the penis of blood are compressed so that most of the blood entering the penis can not drain out. This engorgement is what brings about an erection.

After ejaculation, the accumulated blood flows out of the penis, which then regains its normal size in a flaccid state.

It is interesting to note that upon ejaculation, the nervous system closes the orifice between the urethra and the bladder, preventing semen from mixing with urine and vice versa.

TYPES OF ERECTION

There are three kinds of erection apart from those that result from sexual activity:

- **Reflex erections, common among children and babies, are involuntary and occur without sexual stimulation. Among adults, they can be brought on by rubbing clothes or simply by the vibration of a moving vehicle. Because this type of erection is controlled by a nerve centre at the base of the spine and requires no input from the brain, men with spinal injuries that have not affected this area may get reflex erections.**
- **Psychogenic erections occur when a man has sexual thoughts while watching an erotic film, having amorous thoughts about his partner, or fantasizing.**
- **Nocturnal erections are not well understood, but it is known that healthy men of all ages have three or four erections a night, each one lasting approximately half an hour.**

CROSS-SECTION OF THE PENIS AND CIRCULATORY SYSTEM

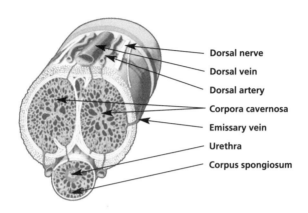

Dorsal nerve
Dorsal vein
Dorsal artery
Corpora cavernosa
Emissary vein
Urethra
Corpus spongiosum

■ TESTOSTERONE IS NOT SYNONYMOUS WITH SEX DRIVE

Testosterone is the primary male hormone or androgen. It is present as the male embryo develops, but its activity is not particularly pronounced until the onset of puberty. At this stage, it is responsible for a young man's deepening voice, the growth of body hair, the development of his muscles and the maturation of his testicles.

Testosterone is also necessary for sexual activity. In fact, its primary role in the adult male is to increase his sexual appetite. The amount of testosterone in the body therefore has an influence on the libido: the man with no testosterone has very little or even no interest in sex.

"But be careful! This does not mean that testosterone is synonymous with sex drive. Interest in sex depends on a number of other factors: education, age, the man's personality, his partner's personality, the couple's particular situation, and so on. In fact, all aspects of a man's life can affect his sexual desire. Hormones are not everything!" emphasizes Dr. McCormack. Testosterone will be discussed further in the section on andropause in chapter 2.

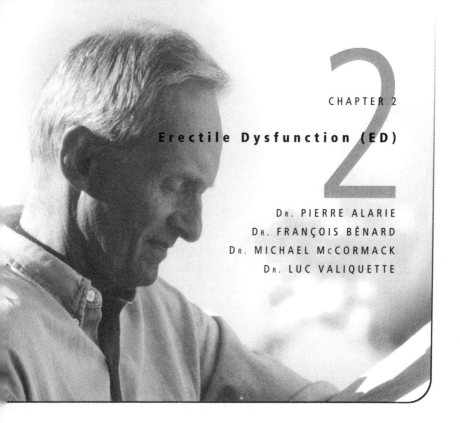

Erectile Dysfunction (ED)

Dr. PIERRE ALARIE
Dr. FRANÇOIS BÉNARD
Dr. MICHAEL McCORMACK
Dr. LUC VALIQUETTE

▨ WHAT EXACTLY IS ERECTILE DYSFUNCTION ?

Erectile dysfunction is defined as a persistent inability to achieve or maintain an erection adequate for satisfying sexual intercourse. Now perceived to be pejorative and demeaning, the term "impotence" is no longer used. Erectile dysfunction can manifest in the following ways:

- ▨ difficulty attaining or inability to achieve an erection;
- ▨ erections that are too soft for penetration;
- ▨ inability to maintain the erection after penetration;
- ▨ inability to maintain the erection long enough to achieve orgasm.

This type of problem is very common: according to the Massachusetts Male Aging Study (see frame, page 26), 52% of men between the ages of 40 and 70 experience ED. Younger men can also suffer from it, though the occurrence is less frequent and few statistics are available. Of course, erectile dysfunction is a chronic problem and the occasional case (brought on, for example, by a particularly hard day at work) should be treated as an isolated incident.

"The clinical guidelines indicate that the problem must last at least three months before erectile dysfunction can be diagnosed. However, a man does not have to wait that long before he consults a doctor. He should make an appointment as soon as it starts to worry him," emphasizes Dr. McCormack.

A man who is not able to achieve penetration can still get sexually aroused, have orgasms and ejaculate. Because erection is generally expected to be a normal part of sexual response, however, erectile dysfunction is considered to be an abnormality and can have serious emotional repercussions.

"In fact, erectile dysfunction affects the mind as much as the body. A man's emotional health and self-perception can impact his physical condition and his sexual performance. Let me explain. When a problem occurs – for physical, psychological, or a combination of the two reasons – a vicious circle can be created. The fear of no longer being able to have 'normal' erections can lead to performance

AN INSTRUCTIVE STUDY

The Massachusetts Male Aging Study (MMAS) provides a wealth of information for doctors and sex therapists. Between 1987 and 1997, the National Institute on Aging in Boston followed 1709 Americans, aged 40 to 70. Spanning ten years, the study has greatly increased the amount of knowledge available about men's general and sexual health.

Among other things, the study showed that erectile dysfunction affected 52% of the participants:

- 17% experienced occasional problems;
- 25% experienced intermittent problems;
- 10% dealt with the problem frequently.

anxiety (where a man has doubts about his virility and capacity as a lover), which only aggravates the situation. As a result, a lot of men just withdraw. Widowers and single men, for example, sometimes stop going out in order to avoid running the risk of meeting someone and having to face their problems in bed. These problems can also have an impact on a couple's relationship. The man's partner may feel less attractive to him and even suspect infidelity.

"There is a lot left to learn about erectile dysfunction, but we do know that, for the most part, it does not happen all of a sudden. On the contrary, it is something that grows more pronounced over time," continues Dr. McCormack. "Erectile dysfunction may occur rarely in the first years, become intermittent after a few more ('sometimes it works, sometimes it doesn't'), and only eventually become chronic."

Is it directly linked to age? "No, it's not that simple. With age, sexual desire may decrease while the amount of stimulation necessary to achieve orgasm increases. This is simply because the body is getting older and slowing down. It is perfectly normal and doesn't stop a couple from having mutually satisfying sexual relations. In other words, not being as frisky at 70 as you were at 20 doesn't mean you're suffering from erectile dysfunction!"

Erectile dysfunction is not inevitable. It does not occur in all men of a certain age. Furthermore, the MMAS study indicates that

CAN A MAN HAVE ERECTILE PROBLEMS FOR NO REASON?

Yes, it is possible, but the vast majority of patients have at least one risk factor, either physical or psychological.

A man who is in good shape, in love, and happy with his life should not experience erectile dysfunction. If he does, there is almost always an underlying reason that either a doctor or sex therapist can help him discover.

52% of men between 40 and 70 have erectile problems, which also means that 48% of them have preserved their powers! If erectile dysfunction is more common in older men, it is because these men are more likely to have underlying health conditions that can cause the problem.

There are several risk factors that can contribute to erectile dysfunction: vascular disease (blood vessel problems), neurological disorders (nerve damage), psychological problems, conditions directly related to the penis, endocrine disorders (hormone imbalances), certain drugs, and life-style habits. It should also be noted that erectile difficulties can sometimes happen for no apparent reason.

"Often, or I should even say most of the time, there is more than one causal factor," points out Dr. McCormack. "Suppose an obese smoker with diabetes and high blood pressure comes to my office. His erectile difficulties, on top of everything else, have probably also given him performance anxiety. Because the combination of these factors is responsible for his erectile dysfunction, it is not always possible to determine a single cause with precision, which is why doctors prefer to talk about risk factors. The more risk factors appear, the higher the chance of erectile dysfunction."

Erectile dysfunction can also be a symptom of an underlying illness. For example, a man who is suffering from erectile difficulties because of arteriosclerosis (hardening of the arteries) in the penis is also likely to be suffering from arteriosclerosis in his other arteries. In this case, erectile dysfunction is a reflection of a more generalized vascular disease. Another good reason to see your doctor!

■ CAUSES OF ERECTILE DYSFUNCTION

An erection is the result of an engorgement of blood in the cavernous bodies of the penis. It is a vascular process involving the neurological system, the hormones, and the psyche. Any of the factors or disorders listed below can interfere in some way with its complicated mechanics.

VASCULAR DISEASES
- Arteriosclerosis (hardening of the arteries)
- Heart disease
- High cholesterol
- High blood pressure
- Kidney and hepatic (liver) failure
- Diabetes

NEUROLOGICAL DISORDERS
- Diabetes
- Multiple sclerosis
- Spinal cord injuries
- Pelvic (lower abdominal) trauma
- Alzheimer's disease
- Parkinson's disease
- Stroke
- Spina bifida

PSYCHOLOGICAL PROBLEMS
- Depression
- Performance anxiety
- Stress
- Psychosis

CONDITIONS RELATING TO THE PENIS
- Peyronie's disease
- Priapism
- Congenital malformations

ENDOCRINE PROBLEMS

- Diabetes
- Hypogonadism
- Hyperprolactinemia
- Hyperthyroidism
- Hypothyroidism
- Andropause

MEDICATIONS

- Hypoglycaemic drugs
- Antihypertensives (for high blood pressure)
- Antidepressants
- Antipsychotic drugs
- Anticonvulsive drugs
- Tranquillizers
- Antihistamines

LIFE-STYLE HABITS

- Smoking
- Alcoholism
- Drug addiction
- Extreme obesity

DIABETES

Why devote an entire section to this condition? Because it has long been known that diabetes is the most common cause of erectile dysfunction. In fact, about 40% of men with erectile difficulties also suffer from diabetes. The reason these conditions so often overlap is that diabetes is a very common disease – affecting 7% of the population – and impacts nearly all elements of the erection mechanism, from the vascular and neurological systems to the hormones.

Diabetes is a chronic disease characterized by the body's inability to process sugar. It is linked to insulin, a hormone secreted by the pancreas, which is a gland in the digestive tract. Insulin allows glucose to enter the cells for use and storage. Diabetes develops if the pancreas stops producing insulin (type 1), or if the body resists the production and action of insulin (type 2). In both types, excessive amounts of unprocessed leftover sugar remain in the blood (hyperglycaemia) and urine.

In addition to erectile dysfunction, both type 1 and 2 diabetes have the following symptoms: excessive thirst, frequent urination (to the point of disturbing sleep), rapid breathing, unexplained weight loss, genital itchiness, bad vision, extreme fatigue and, in more advanced stages, partial and progressive numbness of the feet.

"Ten percent of diabetics suffer from type 1, which is particularly prevalent in children and young adults. It develops in genetically predisposed people when a trigger, such as a viral infection, activates the body's immune system to begin destroying the beta cells of the pancreas, which are necessary for the production of insulin. The symptoms are the same, but more severe than those of type 2 diabetes. For the type 1 sufferer, erectile difficulties usually begin quite early in life, around the age of thirty. A man with type 1 diabetes, therefore, usually suffers from ED longer than the type 2 diabetic," explains Dr. Alarie.

Type 2 diabetes generally affects people over 40 years of age and is caused by an unhealthy lifestyle (obesity, sedentary habits, consumption of excessive amounts of fatty foods). Genetics are also a factor: people whose parents had type 2 diabetes are twice as likely to develop it themselves. In many cases, early symptoms are so mild that many sufferers fail to even notice them, remaining unaware of their disease for a number of years.

HOW DOES DIABETES HAMPER ERECTION?

Too much sugar in the blood causes the blood vessels to harden and thicken. This loss of elasticity prevents the blood vessels of the penis from dilating enough to fill the cavernous bodies. When less blood flows into the penis, the cavernous bodies cannot effectively constrict the veins that allow blood to flow out. This causes a venous leak whereby the blood seeps out of the penis, making it more difficult to reach and maintain erection.

An excess of sugar in the blood also destroys the sheath around the nerve endings and prevents impulses from travelling along nerves that control erection. Thus, messages from the brain and spinal cord do not reach the penis. High blood sugar also reduces the levels of certain chemicals necessary for erection (such as nitric oxide).

Diabetes also causes kidney problems that can develop into kidney failure. In this case, an excessive amount of urea – a waste product that is usually flushed out with the urine – remains in the body and affects the entire nervous system, including those nerves essential to erection.

A decrease in testosterone has also been noted in diabetic men. Some research has shown lower levels of this male hormone in 21% of diabetic men, compared to 13% of other men in the same age bracket. It is also known that the less balanced the blood sugar levels, the more pronounced the drop in testosterone. The body may even stop producing testosterone altogether if the patient does not correctly manage his diabetes. Fortunately, testosterone levels and sexual desire return to normal when the disease is once again under control.

If all of these complications were not enough, diabetes can also cause premature, delayed or retrograde ejaculation (*see chapter 3*), as well as a fairly unique problem known as dribbling ejaculation, whereby the semen trickles down the length of the penis instead of being forcefully expelled. This is caused by a malfunction of the nerves that regulate the two muscles responsible for semen expulsion, located at the base of the penis. This condition occurs in about 10% of diabetics.

AN INSIDIOUS DISEASE

The patient with diabetes (either type 1 or 2) will often develop erectile dysfunction in the early stages of the disease. For a large proportion of diabetics, in fact, ED is the first symptom. Researchers have also found that some men even start having difficulties with erection while suffering from glucose intolerance (the phase preceding diabetes).

"By the age of 50, about half of diabetic men suffer from erectile dysfunction; by age 70, 95% do. With age, other elements like hypercholesterolemia, smoking, or high blood pressure make the situation worse," emphasizes Dr. Alarie. "The more diabetes progresses, the more damage it does. A diabetic man's erectile dysfunction will get worse and worse, often to the point where it becomes impossible for him to get an erection."

What happens if the disease is controlled well? "Certainly, if a man with type 1 or 2 diabetes manages his condition properly, some damage to the erection mechanism can be prevented, especially if

CASE STUDY

JOHN AND HIS DIABETES

John is 68 years old and has been diabetic since the age of 42. He balances his cholesterol through diet, and quit smoking fifteen years ago. He consults his family doctor every six months, and at every visit, his blood pressure is normal.

Over the last three years, he has experienced erectile dysfunction with increasing frequency and his wife is starting to become worried. So is he, in fact, since he only lacks ability, not desire. Although he has always been too shy to do so in the past, he finally decides to broach the subject with his doctor.

The doctor listens to John's story, conducts an examination, and determines that the erectile dysfunction is due to diabetes. He explains that diabetes is an insidious disease affecting the cardiovascular, neurological and hormonal systems, all of which are central to the mechanism of erection. Furthermore, even though John quit smoking years ago, the permanent damage it did to his arteries is now likely contributing to the ED. The doctor takes this opportunity to remind John of the importance of managing his diabetes through diet, and they discuss the use of a blood sugar calendar to help him control the disease. They also consider the possibility of specific treatments for his ED.

the disease is diagnosed early. Medical treatment, however, will not necessarily make lesions on the blood vessels or nerves disappear. The erectile problem can sometimes be stabilized, but we can't promise men that they will function exactly as they used to."

While type 1 can be more easily detected because it affects children and young adults, 50% of those with type 2 diabetes remain unaware of their condition for a prolonged period. This is a serious problem. "If men notice changes in their erections or a few mild symptoms, they do not necessarily make the connection to diabetes. They chalk it up to fatigue or something else and only find themselves at the doctor's office once their health has seriously deteriorated – for example, when they are experiencing numbness in their feet, a sign that the disease has already progressed to an advanced stage."

■ VASCULAR DISEASES

As we saw in chapter 1, erection occurs when the cavernous bodies of the penis are engorged with blood. If circulation to the blood vessels of the penis is poor, therefore, problems are inevitable.

According to the Massachusetts Male Aging Study (MMAS), 44% of men with heart disease also suffer from complete erectile dysfunction. Compare this figure to the mere 9% of men without heart disease who suffer the same.

"The build-up of cholesterol in the blood vessels, or arterio-sclerosis, is the primary impediment to blood circulation. Over time, cholesterol deposits obstruct the arteries and cause them to lose their elasticity," explains Dr. Valiquette.

We know about the dangers arteriosclerosis poses to the coronary arteries: angina pectoris, myocardial infarction (heart attack) and heart failure. What we often forget, however, is that arteriosclerosis also blocks other blood vessels, such as those of the penis. These are, in fact, particularly vulnerable to obstruction because of their small diameter. If the blockage is significant enough to prevent blood from accumulating in the cavernous bodies, erectile dysfunction will ensue.

Initially, vessel obstruction causes partial erections. Although the patient can still get an erection, they are either more difficult to achieve and maintain, or insufficiently firm. Over the years, as the vascular disease progresses, the blood vessels become more obstructed and erectile dysfunction more pronounced. Blood circulation, in fact, can eventually slow to a virtual halt, making erection impossible. ED is then complete.

Other vascular diseases can have a negative impact on erection capacity. Arterial hypertension (high blood pressure) causes the heart and blood vessels to work extra hard and the walls of the blood vessels to harden or contract. Diabetes can also eventually cause blood vessel blockage, especially if the disease is poorly managed. Hypercholesterolemia (high cholesterol) is risky, as well: the higher the levels of blood cholesterol, the higher the chances of cholesterol deposits on blood vessel walls. High cholesterol usually leads to arteriosclerosis if left untreated. And it should be stressed again that since these diseases affect not only the blood vessels in the penis, but also cause damage to the coronary arteries that could lead to heart disease, they should never be taken lightly.

"I often tell my patients that the penis is a mirror of the heart, and vice versa. If blood circulation in the penis is poor, it often indicates a more generalized vascular disease that may also be affecting the coronary arteries. Similarly, if a patient is suffering from heart disease and the coronary arteries are either partially or completely blocked, it is very likely that the blood vessels in the penis will be blocked, as well. This is why erection problems are so common in patients with a history of heart disease. Several studies have shown that the rate of heart disease is higher in men with erectile dysfunction, and vice versa. The connection is not automatic, but the two problems often coincide," says Dr. Valiquette

Several medications (such as those for high blood pressure) that act on the cardiovascular system can also have a negative impact on erectile function. Chronic kidney failure and liver failure, furthermore, cause imbalances such as high blood pressure and high cholesterol, which lead to erectile difficulties.

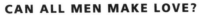

CAN ALL MEN MAKE LOVE?

About 2% of men are not able to have sexual relations because of their heart conditions.

Sexual activity and orgasm increase the heart rate to 120 or 130 beats per minute (the normal rate is 72), and significantly raise blood pressure. Basically, making love is like running up two flights of stairs, lifting a 20-pound weight, or playing 18 holes of golf while carrying your own bag!

If a man cannot perform these activities without becoming exhausted or having an angina attack, he may be at risk of having a heart attack while making love. Note that this warning does not apply to men who quickly lose their breath when climbing stairs. Respiratory difficulties caused by smoking, emphysema or pulmonary insufficiency, for example, do not put men at the same risk.

Men with heart disease, or those who have suffered a heart attack or undergone heart surgery (bypass or angioplasty, for example) must speak to their doctors about their capacity to have sexual relations.

It is also important to note that making love less than three hours after eating, after drinking alcohol, or during very hot weather requires more energy and increases the risk of heart attack. Furthermore, it seems that extramarital affairs are also bad for the heart, probably because the man is trying to outdo himself sexually – or perhaps because he is afraid of getting caught!

Can a man with heart disease take sildenafil (Viagra)? Yes, he can, as long as he is not taking any nitrate based medications and his doctor says his heart is strong enough for him to have sexual relations.

■ NEUROLOGICAL CONDITIONS

The dilation of blood vessels in the penis necessary for erection is controlled by nerves, damage to which may lead to erectile dysfunction. The key nerves are not only located in the genital area, but also run through the spinal column, connecting the brain to the penis.

The neurological complications of diabetes (resulting from poor management of blood sugar levels), spinal cord injury, multiple sclerosis and injuries to the pelvic area are the most common ways nerves that control erection are damaged.

SPINAL CORD INJURY

Surgery or back injury may cause spinal cord trauma that damages or destroys the nerve circuits controlling erection. Some men who

INJURY AT NECK LEVEL

The nerves responsible for psychogenic erection branch off from the spinal cord at the thoracic level (T11, T12) and the lumbar level (L1, L2).

The nerves responsible for reflex erections branch off from the spinal cord at the sacral level (S2, S3, S4).

T11 to L2

Result: loss of psychogenic erections, but reflex erections are still possible.

Sacral level S2 to S4

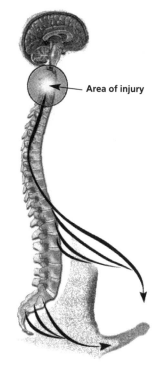

Area of injury

have had surgery close to the spinal column may experience complications in the form of temporary or permanent erectile dysfunction, depending on the severity of the injury to the spinal cord. Complications from surgery on a herniated disk, for example, or postoperative bleeding that injures the spinal cord or certain nerve roots, can lead to ED.

It can also occur in men whose spinal column has been injured or severed in an accident. Paraplegics (those paralysed below the waist, in two limbs) or quadriplegics, also known as tetraplegics (those paralysed below the neck, in all four limbs), generally have no feeling in their genital organs.

Does this mean they can never have erections? "It depends on the severity of the injury to the spinal cord," responds

LOWER BACK INJURY

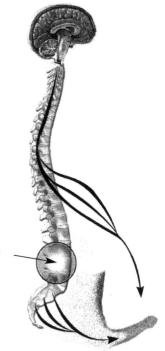

Lower back injury below L2 and above sacral spinal cord (S2, S3, S4).

Result: both types of erection are still possible.

T11 to L2

Area of injury

Sacral level S2 to S4

Dr. Valiquette. "If the injury is not complete – that is, if some of the nerve fibres in the spinal cord remain intact – the man may be able to recover a measure of his former erection capacity. If the spinal cord is completely severed, however, the patient will lose control of his erections and no longer be able to ejaculate, even though he may still have reflex erections. "

Reflex erections do not depend on the brain, but on the nerve complex that controls these reflexes, located near the base of the spinal column, around the level of the navel. If the spinal cord injury occurs above this centre, contact between the brain and the genitals is severed. Since the nerve complex remains intact, however, the patient will still get reflex erections. Unfortunately, these erections cannot be controlled, are of variable duration,

INJURY TO SACRAL SPINAL CORD

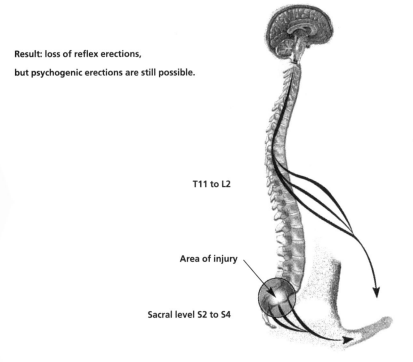

Result: loss of reflex erections,
but psychogenic erections are still possible.

T11 to L2

Area of injury

Sacral level S2 to S4

CAN A PARALYSED MAN START A FAMILY?
Only 10% to 20% of men with spinal cord injuries
are able to have sex and ejaculate without
treatment.

For the other 80% or so, while erectile function can be salvaged with drugs like sildenafil (Viagra), recovering the capacity to ejaculate is more complicated. This requires medically-assisted techniques such as stimulating the glans with vibration (used in fertility clinics), or injecting drugs into the spinal column.

In many cases, the couple must resort to medically-assisted reproduction.

and produce no pleasure for the man since contact with the brain has been cut off.

"The erections most men with spinal cord injuries have are not reliable enough for satisfying sex, which is very tragic since these injuries often happen to young men (in car, motorcycle or skiing accidents, for example). The impact on the man's sex life is permanent and very difficult to deal with. Fortunately, there are a number of medical treatments available that can produce firm, reliable erections and make sexual relations possible again."

MULTIPLE SCLEROSIS

Twice as many women as men suffer from multiple sclerosis, which is a chronic neurological disease that can affect various parts of the body and manifest differently from one person to the next. Early symptoms include difficulty enunciating, vision problems, loss of balance, extreme fatigue, and more often than not, erectile difficulties. According to certain studies, 75% of men with this disease suffer from sexual dysfunction, which is brought on by damage both to the protective myelin sheath around the spinal cord, and to the nerves that carry messages from the brain to the genitals.

People with multiple sclerosis suffer symptoms episodically and with varying intensity, enjoying periods of remission during which the man may recover all of his sexual capacity. Unfortunately, as the disease progresses, so does the erectile dysfunction. Eventually, as the sufferer becomes so neurologically handicapped that he requires a wheelchair for mobility, erection will no longer be possible.

INJURIES TO THE PELVIC (LOWER ABDOMINAL) AREA

Operations on the intestines, colon, or rectum (for the treatment of cancer or inflammatory bowel diseases such as ulcerous colitis or Crohn's disease) can bring about erectile disorders if they damage the nerves of the pelvic area. The same may occur during lower abdominal surgery to treat aneurysms (the dilation of an artery) or stenosis (blocked arteries). The operation that most commonly causes erectile dysfunction, however, is radical prostatectomy (the removal of the prostate and seminal vesicles for the treatment of

POSSIBLE DAMAGE DUE
TO PROSTATE CANCER SURGERY

(SIMPLIFIED DIAGRAM)

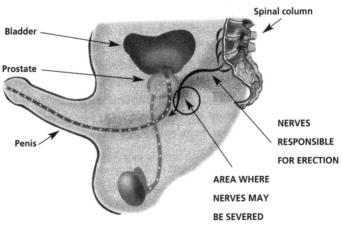

Spinal column

Bladder

Prostate

Penis

NERVES
RESPONSIBLE
FOR ERECTION

AREA WHERE
NERVES MAY
BE SEVERED

prostate cancer). Radical prostatectomies and transurethral prostatectomies must be differentiated. The latter, often resorted to as treatment for benign prostate hypertrophy, involves the excision of a section of the prostate using special instruments that pass through the urethra. Although medications are increasingly used to treat this condition, it is still a relatively common procedure that, unlike radical prostatectomy, does not frequently cause erectile difficulties.

After undergoing a radical prostatectomy for prostate cancer, at least 50% of men suffer from erectile dysfunction. "About twenty years ago, nearly 100% of men had erection problems after this operation, but the numbers have gone down thanks to improved surgical techniques that protect the nerves and blood vessels responsible for erection," explains Dr. Valiquette. Men under the age of 50, furthermore, have a better chance of recovering their erectile function than older men, probably because their blood vessels are in better shape.

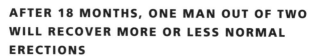

AFTER 18 MONTHS, ONE MAN OUT OF TWO WILL RECOVER MORE OR LESS NORMAL ERECTIONS

About one-third of men with prostate cancer will undergo radical prostatectomy.

One month after the operation, few men will be able to achieve erection, regaining their erectile capacity only little by little.

After 18 months, approximately one man out of two will have recovered his capacity for erection without medication. Nearly half of the others will resort to sildenafil (Viagra), the rest of the patients choosing another form of treatment.

Of course, because the prostate gland and seminal vesicles have been removed, the body can no longer produce semen. While this makes ejaculation impossible, the men may still enjoy the sensation of orgasm.

Radiation therapy (irradiation with radioactive waves) in the pelvic area is often used to treat prostate cancer, which may also cause ED. "Unlike radical prostatectomy, however, radiation therapy does not affect erectile function immediately. As soon as the man begins to feel better, he can take up his normal sexual activities again. Because radiation therapy burns tissues and nerves gradually, erectile dysfunction takes time to appear, but after five years, at least 50% will suffer ED. Chemotherapy, unfortunately, is not considered to be a very effective alternative treatment."

An injury to the pelvic area (for example, if a man's lower body is crushed in a car accident), of course, can also lead to erectile dysfunction, but depending on the severity of the injuries, it is possible that the man will regain full erectile capacity in time.

OTHER NEUROLOGICAL CAUSES

Cerebrovascular events (strokes) can damage the nerve circuit controlling erection. The severity of the erectile dysfunction will depend upon the severity of the stroke. Some men recover their sexual capacity naturally, while others require medical treatment to achieve satisfying erections.

Alzheimer's disease and Parkinson's disease are chronic, degenerative pathologies. They are incurable and gradually worsen to the point of depriving the sufferer of all autonomy. One of the effects of these diseases is damage to the central nervous system, which of course has an impact on the nerves controlling erection. By the time ED appears, however, the disease has usually progressed to such a stage that the man is barely aware of it. As a result, it is not quite accurate to say that he "suffers" from the dysfunction.

Spina bifida (a Latin name meaning "fissured or split spine") is a congenital malformation of unknown origin. This disease causes irreversible and permanent damage to the spinal cord and, in turn, the nervous system. As the disease has varying degrees of severity, so do the erectile difficulties that accompany it.

■ PSYCHOLOGICAL PROBLEMS

DEPRESSION

Depression has the following symptoms: loss of interest in regular activities, withdrawal from social interaction, diminished sexual desire, sleep disorders (insomnia or hypersomnia), weight gain or loss, low energy, difficulty concentrating, feelings of guilt, and morbid and suicidal thoughts. It is a genuine disease, affecting 18% of the population (approximately 8% men) at some point in their lives, and can last several months or even years if left untreated.

Depression is frequently associated with erectile dysfunction. From data recently compiled on his patients, Dr. Alarie found that of the 2000 men suffering from erectile difficulties, 42% showed signs of depression. Official statistics say that 90% of men suffering from serious depression have ED. The two conditions are closely linked, with depression having the potential to bring on erectile dysfunction and, conversely, erectile dysfunction having the potential to cause depression.

It is easy enough to understand why a man suffering from ED might become depressed. But how can depression stop a man from getting an erection? "Basically, it wipes out his sex drive. Despite himself, a depressed man has very little desire to make love and therefore has trouble responding to another's sexual advances. This in turn brings on performance anxiety, or the belief that he will not be able to satisfy his partner," explains Dr. Alarie. "The anxiety triggers an increase in adrenaline, a chemical that causes the blood vessels to constrict. This prevents the dilation of the blood vessels in the penis, thus short-circuiting erection.

"Most of the time, it is very difficult to determine whether depression caused the ED, or the other way around. After a complete medical check-up, the important thing is to treat the two problems together so the patient may recover both a satisfying sex life and mental equilibrium. Both conditions have to be treated as soon as possible; the longer you wait, the worse they get. If the depression worsens, the man runs a serious risk of not being able to achieve erection at all."

Why should both be treated simultaneously? "It's very simple. Most antidepressants cause erectile dysfunction. If we treat only the depression, the ED will continue, the man will not feel he is improving, and then will likely stop taking his medication. Ultimately, he may not even be able to bounce back. On the other hand, if we treat his erectile difficulties without treating his depression, his sex drive will continue to plunge and perpetuate a vicious circle. What's the use, after all, of being able to get an erection if you have no desire to make love!"

Doctors therefore prescribe two types of treatment, one for depression and one for erectile dysfunction. In the vast majority of cases, sildenafil (Viagra) is prescribed. "Occasionally, a man will absolutely refuse to take it because it makes him feel like he has lost his virility, that he's 'not a man' anymore. I explain to them that it's temporary and they need only take it for a few weeks or months."

One study established that 76% of depressed patients experienced

CASE STUDY

BERNARD'S DEPRESSION

Bernard is 47 years old. He is married, the father of two teenagers, and works as a computer scientist. Three months ago, he consulted his doctor for mood swings, insomnia and diminished sex drive.

Upon assessment, the doctor found him to be moderately depressed and prescribed an antidepressant. A few weeks later during a follow-up visit, Bernard told his doctor that he now had erectile problems. The doctor reassured him, explaining that it was a side effect of the medication, and that instead of stopping this treatment, he could prescribe sildenafil (Viagra), as well.

With a slightly bruised ego, Bernard refused at first. He finally understood, however, that if he took sildenafil for only a month or two, his sexual capacity would improve, giving him back his self-confidence and helping him get over his depression.

an improvement in their capacity for erection thanks to Viagra, compared to 18% for those taking placebos. If Viagra does not work, there are other treatments (*see chapter 5*).

Antidepressants are normally prescribed for six to twelve months. "Medical literature recommends using antidepressants for at least a year to ensure the patient makes a complete recovery. Furthermore, we often recommend sex therapy to deal with the psychological consequences of depression and erectile difficulties."

PERFORMANCE ANXIETY

What man, at some point in his life, has not felt that terrible anxiety about failing to satisfy his partner – that fear of falling short?

Any man at any age can suffer from performance anxiety. "If a man focuses too much on his performance, he may not have an erection. He can lose his wherewithal and inadvertently sabotage sexual intercourse," says Dr. McCormack.

Performance anxiety is often experienced by perfectionists who try to outdo themselves in every endeavour, from work, to sports, to raising children. Men who frequently change sexual partners are also at risk, since they generally feel more pressure to perform than those in a stable relationship who enjoy a calmer, more relaxed sex life. Feeling they have to prove themselves to every new conquest night after night, they become overly eager to please and the stress often gets the better of them.

Psychology is obviously a very important factor, but the problem can also be explained physiologically. Fear of failure leads to anxiety and an accompanying burst of adrenaline that causes the blood vessels to constrict (also called vasoconstriction). This prevents the blood vessels from dilating and thereby blocks the erection mechanism.

While performance anxiety can cause erectile dysfunction, it might also be linked to a pre-existing sexual disorder. For example, a man suffering from intermittent erectile disorder ("sometimes it works, sometimes it doesn't") may come to dread his partner's sexual advances. His fear of disappointing his partner can become so intense that anxiety takes over and completely short-circuits his ability to get an erection. Sometimes, all it takes is one episode of erectile dysfunction for performance anxiety to take hold and create a vicious circle (*see frame below*).

Erectile dysfunction and performance anxiety can also cause premature ejaculation. That is, a man dealing with an erectile disorder may become so preoccupied with maintaining his erection that he ejaculates too quickly. Or, conversely, a man may experience performance anxiety because he suffers from premature ejaculation and, as a result, develop erectile dysfunction.

"We have to remember that all sexual disorders – erectile dysfunction, ejaculation problems, diminished desire for sexual intimacy – can co-exist with performance anxiety. In most cases, in fact, they do. If the patient does not deal with both the disorder and the anxiety, the situation will only get worse. Consulting a doctor and a sex therapist can help resolve these issues."

A VICIOUS CIRCLE

Erectile dysfunction episode
▼
Performance anxiety
▼
Next erectile dysfunction episode
▼
Heightened performance anxiety
▼
Decrease in sexual desire
▼
Performance anxiety
▼
Chronic erectile dysfunction

CASE STUDY

BENJAMIN'S PERFORMANCE ANXIETY

Benjamin is a single, 27-year-old professional. His career in computer science is going very well, and keeps him very busy. He is a non-smoker, exercises regularly, eats well, and drinks only when he gets together with friends.

Benjamin and his friends go out to bars every weekend. He meets women on these nights out and frequently ends up spending the night with them. Over the last month, however, Benjamin has not been able to perform in bed with three different partners. Naturally, he is very worried; so much so, in fact, that he is now reluctant to socialize. He is confused about what is happening, and consults his family physician, asking for a complete check-up.

His doctor interviews him about other aspects of his social and professional life to determine whether he is experiencing high levels of stress, but finds that he is not. He asks him if he has morning erections and masturbates, both of which Benjamin confirms. The doctor finds no sign of depression, and everything else seems normal.

The doctor reassures him, explaining that Benjamin is probably suffering from performance anxiety, something that all men encounter at some point in their lives. He advises Benjamin not to take it too seriously, or even think about it at all, if he can, for this is the best way to make the anxiety disappear and set things to rights. In case the problem persists beyond the next few weeks, however, the doctor gives him the name and number of a sex therapist.

STRESS

Stress is a state of anxiety precipitated by an event (job loss, moving, financial problems, trouble at work or with children, etc.). It is much more common than depression, but less serious since it lasts for a shorter period of time. It too, however, can lead to erectile dysfunction. Stress causes an increase in the production of adrenaline – a chemical that causes the blood vessels to contract – which inhibits the dilation of the blood vessels in the penis and thereby prevents erection.

"A man experiencing problems at work, for example, may have no desire to make love. Not only that, he may also have trouble getting an erection," explains Dr. Alarie. "If this happens too many times and his partner is not understanding, he can end up with performance anxiety. In this case, even once the stressful event has passed, the performance anxiety will likely continue, creating a vicious circle that is very hard to break. In these cases, therapy with a sex therapist is often recommended to help a man recover his ability to achieve erection."

▪ CONDITIONS AFFECTING THE PENIS

Sometimes, the state of the penis itself prevents the engorgement of blood necessary for erection. This may occur, for example, with Peyronie's disease, complications from priapism (*see chapter 3*), or congenital malformations of the penis.

Damage to the penis can also be sustained through sports injuries. There is also the so-called "fractured penis" (although, of course, there is no bone to break), whereby the erect penis folds in half upon penetration during vigorous sexual relations, tearing the tissues. Any operation on the cavernous bodies, including surgery to correct a curvature of the penis or Peyronie's disease, also runs the risk of causing damage to the penis.

■ ENDOCRINE PROBLEMS

Diabetes, hypogonadism, hyperthyroidism and hypothyroidism are all endocrine problems that may cause erectile dysfunction. Diabetes results from a misuse of sugar by the pancreas, a gland located behind the stomach. Hypogonadism (of which andropause is one form) is a common condition with varying causes that is characterized by decreased testosterone production. It may develop because the testicles themselves produce less testosterone, which can be the case if the man had the mumps during adolescence or as an adult, or if he suffered trauma to the testicles (for example, due to cancer, or exposure of the genitals to extreme heat). Hypogonadism can also be caused by the malfunction of a gland in the brain called the hypophysis, which results from either prolactinoma (a tumour), or prolactinemia, the over-production of prolactin, a testosterone-reducing hormone produced by the hypophysis.

In addition to erectile dysfunction and loss of sexual desire, the most serious cases of hypogonadism also cause atrophy of the testicles (they become smaller), a decrease in hair growth, and gynecomasty (abnormal growth of the mammary glands in men).

Hyperthyroidism and hypothyroidism are less common risk factors for ED. In both cases, there is an imbalance in the thyroid gland, which is located in the neck: hyperthyroidism results in the over-production of hormones; hypothyroidism, in the under-production. Researchers have determined that these endocrine problems may cause erectile dysfunction, but have not yet understood why.

■ MEDICATIONS

Certain hypoglycemic agents, antihypertensives, antidepressants, antipsychotics, anticonvulsants, tranquillizers and antihistamines can also have a negative effect on erection, although the reasons are not yet fully understood. "We know that antihypertensives lower arterial pressure, affecting the blood that flows to the penis and therefore the extent to which the cavernous bodies can become engorged. We also know that other drugs, like antipsychotics, can affect erection by acting on the transmission of nerve impulses," says Dr. Valiquette. "The active mechanisms of other medications are still unknown. But clearly, taking drugs with the possible side effect of erectile dysfunction increases the risk of suffering from it."

Drug treatment for prostate cancer can also cause erectile dysfunction. Since the progression of prostate cancer is actually encouraged by the presence of testosterone, doctors often prescribe drugs that block the secretion of testosterone (LHRH analogs) or inhibit its action on the cells (antiandrogens). Unfortunately, as the treatment progresses, sexual desire and the ability to become erect are eventually eliminated. "It should also be mentioned that some doctors find it necessary to remove the testicles (castration or orchidectomy), in which case sexual desire and capacity are also lost.

"If a man has been having erectile problems since he first started taking a certain drug, he should ask his pharmacist or doctor if the medication might be causing it. The patient should not, however, stop taking the drug without consulting his doctor, who may choose to change the prescription or reduce the dosage to help deal with any erectile problem. For example, the dosage of high blood pressure medication can be reduced or even stopped if the patient watches his weight, reduces his salt intake, learns how to relax, does light exercise, and follows all of the doctor's other orders. Of course, this must be done under medical supervision."

Sometimes, even if the patient stops taking the drug or replaces it with another medication, he may continue to suffer from erectile dysfunction because he has developed performance anxiety. In this case, a sex therapist should be consulted.

■ CAN LIFESTYLE NEGATIVELY AFFECT SEXUAL ACTIVITY?

The effects of tobacco on the heart are well-known. Smoking causes arteriosclerosis (a narrowing of the coronary arteries) and damage to the endothelium, the inner lining of the blood vessels. Circulation in the coronary arteries is hampered, as it is in the blood vessels of the penis, which are smaller and very easily blocked by the effects of cigarette toxins, thus creating the potential for erectile dysfunction.

"Smoking acts on two levels. When you light a cigarette, the smoke and other toxins have instantaneous effects on the circulatory system: the veins and arteries contract, including those in the cavernous and spongy bodies of the penis, negatively affecting erection. Over the years, furthermore, smoking causes arteriosclerosis, which hinders circulation in the penis," explains Dr. Valiquette. "Studies have shown that smokers suffer from erectile dysfunction two or three times more often than non-smokers. If a man stops smoking, the damage will stop progressing

5 CIGARETTES/DAY = ERECTION PROBLEMS

Scientific studies have shown that smoking only five cigarettes a day can have significant effects on your health, particularly erectile capacity.

A study presented at the American Heart Association's Annual Conference on Cardiovascular Disease Epidemiology and Prevention reveals that men who smoke up to 10 cigarettes a day are 16% more likely to experience erectile dysfunction than non-smokers. Men sho smoke 11 to 20 cigarettes a day have a 36% higher likelihood, and those who smoke more than 20 increase their risk by 60%.

And these negative effects cannot be mitigated by smoking light or menthol cigarettes. Although the toxins in them are less concentrated, people who smoke light cigarettes generally smoke more, and inhale more deeply. In the end, the risks are the same.

and can sometimes repair itself, depending on the man's general state of health."

Do pipes and cigars have the same effect? "Cigarette smokers fully inhale smoke consisting of a multitude of toxins (including nicotine, carbon monoxide and benzene, among others), which are absorbed into the blood. Pipe and cigar smokers rarely inhale, except indirectly, which is why their smoking is less likely to lead to erectile dysfunction."

Alcohol and drugs (either soft or hard) act differently. Taken in large quantities, they "put the brain to sleep." When a man is drunk or on drugs, he is not able to make love, just like he is not able to drive a car or function coherently. Over the years, his capacity will continue to diminish. "Severe drug addicts have bad health in general and suffer from a number of disorders, like heart disease, diabetes, hypercholesterolemia, depression – in short, all conditions that add to the risk of erectile dysfunction."

Bad nutrition and a sedentary lifestyle encourage obesity, which often causes high cholesterol and blood sugar levels eventually leading to erectile problems. The consequences of obesity are similar to those of diabetes; in fact, the former frequently brings on the latter.

■ ANDROPAUSE: MYTH OR REALITY?

Many wonder if andropause (or male menopause) even exists. Although a large number believe it does, it is still highly controversial within the medical community. Magazine articles about how to deal with this stage of life are being published regularly, but doctors cannot yet agree on whether or not it is a real phenomenon.

What is andropause, exactly? "It is an abnormal decrease in testosterone due to an imbalance in the hypophysis, a gland in the brain, which controls the production of testosterone by the testicles. Andropause occurs in men over 40 and manifests in a variety of ways, including erectile dysfunction," explains Dr. Bénard.

It has been proven that after the age of 40, testosterone levels decrease by 1% per year in all men. It is part of the natural aging process and generally goes more or less unnoticed. As they age, men slow down in their daily activities and become a little less ardent in their sex lives. More sexual stimulation is required, as well as more time to recover between bouts of lovemaking. The natural fact that a man is not as vigorous at the age of 60 as he was at 20 does not prevent him from having a satisfying sex life.

Some men, however, experience more pronounced changes, which a number of doctors attribute to a dramatic decrease in testosterone levels. "After 40, many of the following symptoms can manifest: lack of energy, decreased libido, decreased strength and endurance, melancholia and irritability, difficulty enjoying life, less capacity to engage in regular sports activities, excessive sleepiness after evening meals, hot flashes, erectile dysfunction, trouble concentrating, weight gain in the abdomen and hips ('love handles'), decreased productivity at work,

A HYPOTHESIS SLOWLY GAINING ACCEPTANCE

Spurred in large part by the desire of baby-boomers to hold on to their youth, the theory of andropause was born out of an increasing interest since the 1990s in the changes men undergo as they age.

The World Health Organization (WHO) recognized that the concept was worthy of study and very possibly a real phenomenon in 1998.

Since then, studies have tended to confirm its existence, although it has yet to be proven unequivocally. In the medical and scientific community, 70% of professionals believe it exists, while 30% discount it.

Clear answers should be available soon. Scientists are continuing to study the issue in depth and drawing inevitably closer to determining whether there actually is an abnormal level of testosterone and what it might be.

and lowered bone-density (which can lead to osteoporosis and an increased risk of bone fracture)."

How many men does it affect? "We don't know exactly. Some scientists say that 10% of men are affected; others say 30%. Andropause is a new theory and, unlike menopause, still not considered to be an irrefutable scientific fact. There are no medical markers or criteria to clinically define it. Nor do we know which testosterone level should act as our base-line for measurement. Since levels change with age, it is difficult to say exactly whether a decrease is normal or abnormal, which only adds to the controversy.

"Actually, many doctors just don't believe it exists. Instead, they think the drop in testosterone is inevitable and that symptoms such as erectile dysfunction can spring from a number of other sources: for example, libido problems, fatigue, diabetes, professional burn-out, depression, thyroid problems, obesity, alcohol consumption, or smoking. And most of the time, they are right. Although I personally believe that andropause is a genuine condition, I have found that only 25% of my patients who believe they are experiencing it actually are. It is much less common than menopause, which affects all women without exception," says Dr. Bénard.

WHAT KIND OF TESTOSTERONE?

Can we measure the level of testosterone in a man's body? "Yes, it can be measured in a blood sample, but it is not quite that simple. In a man's body, testosterone exists in three forms: free testosterone, which affects men's energy levels and constitutes 2% of all the testosterone in the body; testosterone bonded to albumin, a blood protein, which acts as an easily-accessible reserve to replace the free testosterone that is used up; and finally, testosterone bonded to a globulin (another type of blood protein), which is also a reserve stock, although less readily available. The two types that significantly affect men's energy and libido are free testosterone and albumin-bonding testosterone, which together are known as bio-available testosterone."

Levels of the other, globulin-bonding type increase with age. When testosterone is measured, a record is made of the global levels, or the total of the three forms of the hormone. The increase in the globulin-bonding type will mask any decline in the level of bio-available testosterone. "This is why a man with all the symptoms of a hormone level drop may be told by his doctor that everything is fine: even if there has been a significant decrease in the level of bio-available testosterone, his global testosterone level may still be normal.

"Let's make an analogy. It's like someone with $1 million in the bank, $50 000 in a safe at home, but only $3 in his pocket. He may seem rich, but he can't really do anything with only $3, just like he can't do much with a low level of bio-available testosterone. This is why doctors who believe in andropause measure the levels of bio-available testosterone and well-informed patients generally insist on this type of test, even though current tools are not adequate to precisely measure the levels."

Whatever the case, a man experiencing the symptoms of andropause should consult a doctor and undergo a complete examination. If all other physical and psychological factors are excluded, and if the doctor believes in andropause, the patient can request a dose of bio-available testosterone. If the doctor is a sceptic, however, the treatment will likely go no further. It will then be up to the patient to claim his test results and consult another doctor, if he wishes.

HORMONE REPLACEMENT THERAPY

When a doctor believes the patient is lacking testosterone, he or she may prescribe hormone replacement therapy, which has a number of benefits, including the recovery of normal levels of energy, muscular strength and self-esteem. It is not, however, a miracle treatment. Because the libido depends on a number of other factors, testosterone supplements will not solve problems in a relationship, or make a man lose any sexual inhibitions he has experienced all his life. The hormone will bring him back to his old self, but will not turn him into a sex machine!

Hormone replacement will also help decrease cholesterol levels, thus preventing cardiovascular diseases. This is a considerable benefit, since the risk of heart disease increases with age. Furthermore, the treatment reduces the risk of osteoporosis and helps promote a general sense of well-being.

Testosterone supplements can be administered in four different ways: by injection, orally, through skin patches or a gel. The least expensive mode is injection, administered intra-muscularly every two to three weeks by the patient himself. "The problem with this method is that the testosterone level sometimes rises excessively immediately following the injection, and drops below normal levels a few days before the next dose."

Pills allow the patient to maintain a more stable testosterone level, since they are taken more regularly, usually two to three times a day (four to six pills). Skin patches, placed on the thigh, chest or shoulder, also provide a steady testosterone level, although they occasionally come off the skin or cause irritation and some men find them unsightly. In 10% of cases, men experience an allergic reaction, forcing them to use another method.

The gel is a new product and is applied on the tops of the shoulders or the chest. "It takes about six hours before the product is fully absorbed. During this period, the man must avoid taking a shower or having direct physical contact. If his female partner touches the gel, she will also absorb the testosterone and very likely suffer ill effects, such as increased body hair and menstruation and fertility problems. A woman must never apply the gel for her partner and the man must always wash his hands and wear a tee-shirt until it is fully absorbed."

All the methods of delivery are equally effective. Injection and pills are the most popular, but are losing some ground to the more recent skin patches and gels. Side effects of hormone therapy are rare, but take the form of acne, high red blood cell count, and increased risk of oedema (swelling). If the man absorbs too much testosterone (if his dosage is incorrect or if he takes more than prescribed), he may even develop the symptoms of severe hypergonadism: testicular atrophy, reduction in body hair and gynecomasty (abnormal growth of mammary glands in men). Too large a quantity of testosterone can cause the body to transform at least some of the male hormone into oestrogen, a female hormone.

"The risk of oedema (which usually occurs in the legs) is dangerous for those suffering from heart failure or uncontrolled high blood pressure; hormone therapy can be contraindicated in these cases. Nor is it recommended for men who have had prostate cancer, since testosterone actually nourishes the cancer. It is also contraindicated for men suffering from breast cancer (a very rare occurrence in men), since this cancer is also stimulated by testosterone."

Can hormone replacement therapy cause cancer in men, as it is now feared it can in women? "No, not as far as we know. Male and female hormone therapy are completely different and should not be compared. The current position in the scientific community is that women's sex hormone levels drop much more dramatically during menopause than men's do during andropause. Since female hormone therapy tries to bring a woman's hormone levels back to where they were before menopause, the amount of hormones they are given is higher, which can lead to undesired consequences.

"However, men should be aware that long term studies on male hormone therapy have yet to be done, since the therapy is quite new. With time and more research, the benefits of hormone replacement therapy for men may be reconsidered. This is why men in hormone treatment are currently followed quite closely by their doctors, consulting every three months for the first year, and then every six months. The doctor pays particular attention to the prostate to be sure no cancer is developing, which would be aggravated by the hormone therapy."

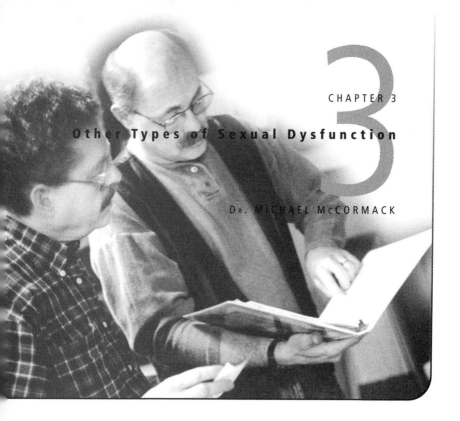

CHAPTER 3

Other Types of Sexual Dysfunction

Dʀ. Michael McCormack

◼ EJACULATION DISORDERS

PREMATURE EJACULATION

Premature ejaculation has been recognized as a genuine sexual disorder since Masters and Johnson published their study of American sexuality in the 1960s. It is one of the most commonly occurring disorders, affecting an estimated 35% of men. "The condition exists when ejaculation occurs too quickly and uncontrollably," explains Dr. McCormack. "The man reaches the point of no return almost immediately nearly every time he makes love. Unable to hold himself back, he ejaculates either before penetration or a few moments after."

Some authors distinguish between primary and secondary premature ejaculation. A man is said to be suffering from primary premature ejaculation when the condition has always existed, and secondary premature ejaculation when he has previously enjoyed a normal sex life.

"Our knowledge of the human body has significantly increased in recent years. We now know, for example, that premature ejaculation is chiefly linked to physiology and does not have a psychological root, as was once believed."

For a number of years, psychological theories were widely accepted explanations for the disorder. "A Freudian theory stated that a man suffered from premature ejaculation because he developed a fear of getting caught in the act during his early sexual experiences. He therefore always unconsciously felt that he had to have an orgasm as quickly as possible, which became a habit and progressively worsened into a chronic problem." Psychoanalysis was recommended in such cases. Other theories placed the blame on problematic sexual development, for which psychotherapeutic treatments like Gestalt, thought stopping, transactional analysis or group therapy were recommended.

EJACULATION
(SIMPLIFIED DIAGRAM)

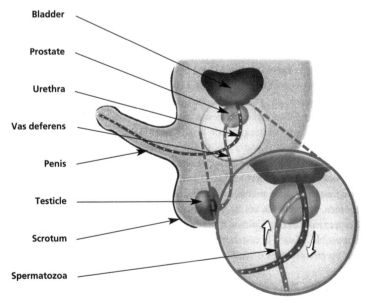

Bladder

Prostate

Urethra

Vas deferens

Penis

Testicle

Scrotum

Spermatozoa

COURSE OF SPERMATOZOA

"The problem," says Dr. McCormack, "is that these theories were based on minimal scientific research or clinical data." Some research now indicates that certain cases of premature ejaculation are due to hypersensitivity of the skin of the penis, and some men find that they can occasionally control their ejaculation by applying an anaesthetic cream to the glans of the penis.

Other research suggests that premature ejaculation is a neurobiological phenomenon (involving cells and nerve tissue), and related to neurotransmitter chemical activity in the brain. For several years now, doctors have been using certain drugs (namely, antidepressants) that act on serotonin, a type of neurotransmitter. They have the effect of delaying ejaculation, and can therefore be used to treat some cases of premature ejaculation. Furthermore, animal research has shown that certain areas of the brain seem to play an important role in ejaculation. As research continues, it will likely soon be possible to identify precisely where in the brain this problem occurs.

It is also known that neurological damage caused by diabetes can affect the nerves of the penis. Among other consequences, this can bring about a premature ejaculation problem. "We have recently learned that genetic factors can also have a significant impact on premature ejaculation. So as you can see, we have moved quite far beyond the psychological theories that were dominant thirty years ago."

Even though physiological factors play a primary role, psychology is still an important element, frequently making the sexual disorder more acute. For example, premature ejaculation can cause a man to

DID YOU KNOW?
According to scientific studies, approximately 90% of men who suffer from premature ejaculation have n orgasm within the first minute of penetration. 80% of these ¬en ejaculate within the first 30 seconds.

develop performance anxiety and lead to problems in the couple's relationship.

"Many men feel a great deal of guilt about this disorder. It is therefore very important for both men and women to understand that it is, above all, a physical problem," emphasizes Dr. McCormack.

CASE STUDY

WILLIAM'S PREMATURE EJACULATION PROBLEM

William is 38 years old, married, and the father of three children. He is a painter and lives in the suburbs with his family. He is experiencing no financial or marital troubles – his only problem is premature ejaculation.

William has suffered from this problem since his first sexual experiences, but it has been getting worse over the last two years. This is very difficult for him to accept because he had expected control of his ejaculations to improve with age. A few years ago, he consulted a sex therapist and tried a few techniques (including compressing the penis), but to no avail. He is very worried that the problem is becoming a serious issue in his marriage because his wife seems less interested in making love than she used to. Unfortunately, however, he has been too afraid to bring the subject up with her.

William confides in his doctor instead. The evaluation questionnaire and complete examination turn up no abnormalities. The doctor informs him that some medications can delay ejaculation and that sex therapists now have new, more effective methods of dealing with the problem. He also strongly advises William to talk to his wife about his worries.

DELAYED EJACULATION

While some men have trouble controlling their orgasm, others have difficulty ever reaching it. This is called delayed or retarded ejaculation. The condition can take different forms and may have always existed or develop suddenly. Delayed ejaculation is likely present if the man:

- ejaculates only if sexual intercourse lasts for an extended period of time (too long for the partner);
- ejaculates only if fellatio or masturbation is performed by the partner;
- ejaculates only if the man masturbates.

"It is normal for ejaculation to take longer as a man gets older. However, certain drugs such as sedatives, antidepressants, amphetamines, alpha-adrenergic inhibitors (for benign prostate hypertrophy) or alcohol, can also bring the problem on. Diabetics may also suffer from this disorder because neurological damage has slowed the ejaculation mechanism."

ANEJACULATION

In extremely rare cases (less than 5%), the man suffers from anejaculation. This means that he ejaculates very rarely, or never. Like delayed ejaculation, this condition may have existed since the man began engaging in sexual activity, or develop suddenly.

Does this mean the man never experiences an orgasm? "Not necessarily. A man's sexual pleasure is at its peak when he achieves orgasm, which coincides with ejaculation. Ejaculation is the physiological reflex and orgasm, the sensation of pleasure. Normally, you can't have one without the other, but sometimes they don't happen at once. For example, spinal injury patients with lesions on their spinal cord can ejaculate, but do not feel any pleasure because contact with the brain has been severed. Conversely, a patient can experience a kind of 'cerebral orgasm,' feeling the sensation of ejaculation without having an erection or actually ejaculating."

"Delayed ejaculation and anejaculation are still terra incognita for doctors," continues Dr. McCormack. "Even though we understand the ejaculation reflex, the factors that prevent it are difficult to pinpoint because they have a lot to do with psychology or little-understood physiological factors. However, we do know that certain medications, especially antidepressants, can hinder the ejaculation mechanism. The effects disappear when the patient stops taking the drug. "

RETROGRADE EJACULATION

This ejaculation disorder, also known as "dry orgasm," is better understood by doctors, although there are still few statistics available. Retrograde ejaculation describes a condition whereby the man has and feels the sensation of an orgasm, but expels no ejaculate. Instead of passing out of the body through the urethra, the semen travels to the bladder where it mixes with the urine and is flushed out. Frequently, the man does not even notice. It should be emphasized that this does not represent a health danger.

The condition can develop if the mechanism that coordinates the closing of the passage between the urethra and the bladder is damaged. This can occur due to surgery (transurethral prostatectomy for benign prostate hypertrophy, or surgery to the vesical neck, for example), or the advanced stages of diabetes (this type of damage occurs in 30% of diabetics). Another possible cause is congenital deformity of the urinary apparatus (not the penis). Certain drugs, such as alpha-adrenergic inhibitors (taken for benign prostate hypertrophy), can also bring the condition on.

■ PEYRONIE'S DISEASE

This unusual disease was first described in France in 1743 by François Gigot de la Peyronie, surgeon for King Louis XV. Peyronie's disease affects four men out of a thousand and is a benign condition. It can occur at any age, although for reasons unknown, is most common among men in their fifties.

Peyronie's disease is characterized by the formation of a fibrous plaque (similar to scar tissue) in the sheath around the cavernous bodies of the penis. This fibrosis, or hard tissue, is more commonly found on the top of the shaft and is discernible to the touch if the penis is palpated in a flaccid state.

The fibrous plaque causes the tissues of the penis to lose some of their elasticity so the penis cannot extend completely and bends during erection. A slight curvature does not inhibit the man's sex life, but can be painful and, in some cases, become so pronounced that intercourse is difficult or even impossible.

It is estimated that 50% of men with this condition also suffer from erectile dysfunction. "For some men, the erection stops where the fibrous plaque begins, leaving the rest of the penis flaccid. In such a case, it is not possible to maintain an erection firm enough for penetration," explains Dr. McCormack.

The causes for Peyronie's disease are still largely unknown, although there are a number of theories. In some cases, for example, the condition is associated with genetic diseases such as Dupuytren's contraction, which is characterized by a loss of elasticity in the tissues of the palm of the hand, and it is therefore believed that genetics may play a role.

"Whatever the cause, it is important to reassure men who have this disease that it is not dangerous. As I tell my patients, it usually presents in acute form for about twelve months, from the time the deformation first appears through its development. It can cause some pain, but unfortunately, the patient has no choice but to live with the disease. Hopefully, the curvature in the penis will not be so pronounced that it prevents him from making love, even if he has to be a little more acrobatic..." The disease will eventually stop

EYRONIE'S
ISEASE

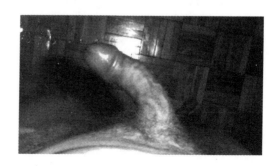

progressing. The extent of the permanent deformation, along with its effects on the man's sex life, will vary. In some men, the penis will return to a nearly normal state with very little deformation, while others will maintain a significant curvature requiring surgery. Since we cannot know in advance how the situation will evolve, the doctor's role is limited to providing information and support to the patient.

CASE STUDY
NORMAN AND HIS EXPERIENCE WITH PEYRONIE'S DISEASE

Norman is a 52-year-old car salesman. He smokes a pack of cigarettes and drinks about three glasses of wine every day, but plays squash several times a week, as well. He got divorced three years ago and is currently seeing someone.

Over the last few months, Norman has noticed a curvature in his penis, that he feels pain during erection, and that the tip of his penis seems to remain soft. All of these symptoms have been making penetration more and more difficult and he is extremely worried. He wants to know what is going on, so consults a doctor.

During the exam, the doctor detects a hard plaque on the underside of the penis that Norman had not noticed. The doctor diagnoses Peyronie's disease and reassures his patient that it is not dangerous, even though the causes are unknown. He refers Norman to a urologist, telling him that he should bring a photograph of his erect penis to show the specialist the extent of the curvature.

The urologist examines the patient and confirms the diagnosis. He prescribes Vitamin E and tells him to come back for a follow-up exam in twelve months. He also reassures Norman that it is not dangerous and that the curvature can be corrected through surgery once the disease has stabilized after about twelve months.

■ PRIAPISM

Unlike Peyronie's disease, priapism is a dangerous condition. Luckily, however, it is also extremely rare. Although it can affect men of any age, even young boys, it is so uncommon that there are no statistics on the problem.

Priapism describes the condition of an erection not brought on by sexual arousal that lasts for more than four hours. It is caused by an abnormal blood flow pattern in the penis, which leads to persistent engorgement and rigidity. It may even occur after ejaculation, if the blood is prevented from flowing back into the body and remains in the penis.

A number of diseases that affect circulation and blood viscosity can cause priapism, such as sickle cell anemia (occurring primarily in black men), diabetes, leukemia and metastasized cancers in the pelvic region. Certain drugs can be responsible, such as anticoagulants, phenothiazines, tradozone, sildenafil (Viagra) and penile injections (see chapter on medical treatments). There have also been cases where priapism occurred when intravenous drug users, having blocked other veins through repeated injections, injected drugs into their penis.

"Priapism can also occur after an injury to the penis or the perineum (the area between the rectum and the testicles). This could happen in a skiing accident, a fight, a football match, or by engaging in extended sexual intercourse with a penis ring."

An emergency doctor should be consulted if the erection lasts for more than four hours. If not treated, the penile tissue can be irreversibly damaged by the formation of a fibrosis, which cannot become engorged with blood for erection. The damage may be so extensive that the man can never achieve erection again. "It should be remembered, however, that although priapism is a serious condition, it doesn't happen out of the blue. Something always causes it," specifies Dr. McCormack.

CASE STUDY
BRIAN'S EXPERIENCE WITH PRIAPISM

Brian is 26 years old and works as a bartender downtown. He has a cocaine habit and although he has tried to quit twice, still buys it and shoots up regularly. The veins of his forearms have become scarred, making injection more difficult recently. Following the suggestion of a friend who is also an addict, Brian injects the drug into his penis.

A few minutes after injecting himself, Brian has an uncontrollable erection. At first he finds it "funny" and "freaky", but six hours later, the erection is still there and starting to become painful. He goes to the emergency room, where the doctor diagnoses priapism and makes an emergency referral to a urologist. The urologist first tries to aspirate blood from the penis, but this has no effect. He then injects an antidote, but it proves to be only temporarily effective, and the priapism soon returns. The urologist then decides to operate and drain the cavernous bodies. Fortunately, the surgery is successful and Brian is able to leave the hospital 24 hours later, suffering no permanent damage.

■ LOWERED SEX DRIVE

Sexual desire, or the libido, is complex. Education, family history, heredity, values, economic situation and social context are among the limitless factors affecting a person's sex drive.

It is perfectly normal if a man does not feel sexually inspired if he has financial problems, for example, or if his child is very sick. Depression, work problems and relationship difficulties can also lead to a lack of desire. He may also have become complacent in his habits. "However, if a man no longer feels excited by his partner, but perks up when he sees his new colleague at work, then some aspect of his relationship is the problem, not his libido," says Dr. McCormack.

Genuine diminished libido occurs for no apparent reason. The man may feel tired and have no desire for any sexual activity whatsoever with anyone at all, but is unable to explain why. Although doctors do not understand the exact causes, they do know that it can become a vicious circle: men experiencing trouble with their sex drive tend to feel anxious about sex. When they do find themselves in an intimate situation, they are usually so worried about not being able to perform that they make little effort. Performance anxiety, detailed in chapter 2, raises its ugly head.

What are the possible causes? "We don't have all the answers. However, we do know that there are certain factors that can contribute to a lowered sex drive: hypogonadism, anemia, diabetes, extreme obesity, a hypophysial (pituitary) tumour, or over-consumption of drugs or alcohol. All of these factors indirectly reduce sexual urges because of fatigue or lowered testosterone. Some also believe that it can be linked to andropause (*see chapter 2*). There are also medications that can inhibit desire, such as antihypertensives, adrenergic receptor inhibitors and finasteride (for benign prostate hypertrophy), antiandrogenes (for prostate cancer), anxiolytic agents, antipsychotics, statin (for high choles-terol), and amphetamines.

Sometimes it is necessary to examine psychological factors, to determine whether the patient is suffering from a sexual phobia (a panicked fear of sex because of fear of commitment, for example), sexual aversion (extreme repugnance to sexual intimacy) or other deep psychological problems. "The patient with no sexual desire is a medical challenge, because there is such a vast range of possible causes. A man suffering from this should consult a doctor to first find out whether an underlying physical problem or drug he is taking may be lowering his sex drive."

CASE STUDY
PETER'S DIMINISHED LIBIDO

Peter is a 57-year-old professor. Usually dynamic and full of vigour, he has noticed a certain loss of energy over the last few months, to the point where he no longer engages in sports activities. His wife complains that he is always tired and makes him feel bad about his lack of sexual appetite. Having heard about andropause and suspecting he may be suffering from it, he decides to consult his doctor.

The doctor finds no specific problem in a general exam, and therefore decides to test the level of bio-available testosterone, which is found to be considerably below normal. To find out why, the doctor also tests prolactin levels, which, if high, may lead to a decrease in testosterone. Because this hormone level is slightly above normal, the doctor suspects a tumour in the hypophysis. Fortunately, however, an endocrinologist verifies that this is not the case. The doctor and Peter then discuss the possibility of hormone replacement therapy to remedy his low levels of testosterone.

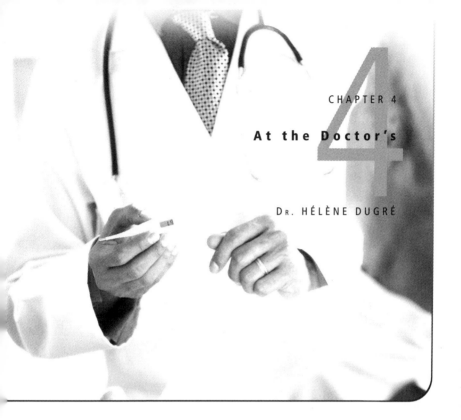

■ CONSULT YOUR DOCTOR

Men are often reluctant to consult a doctor and tend to go only when very worried (or if forced by their partner). It is no different when they are suffering from sexual dysfunction and it may even be worse considering the embarrassment the subject still causes, despite no longer being taboo. This feeling, of course, is perfectly normal, but must be overcome if the problem is to be solved.

The family doctor is the first person to consult. General practitioners are usually well-informed about male sexual disorders and can assess, diagnose and suggest the most appropriate treatment. Moreover, a man's family doctor, familiar with the patient's medical history and psychosocial context, is best able to gather a comprehensive perspective on the problem.

"Some men, however, feel more comfortable talking about their problem with a doctor they don't know and this is perfectly legitimate.

The important thing is to recognize that there is a problem and talk about it if it worries you," emphasizes Dr. Dugré, who, over the years, has learned how to understand what a patient really means when he says, "Doctor, it doesn't work the way it used to..."

It is interesting to note that, since more and more women are entering the medical profession, there will soon be more women in practice than men. Is it difficult for female doctors to talk with their male patients about sexual disorders? And are men more reluctant to consult a female doctor about their problem? "No, it makes no difference at all. I see as many male patients as my male colleagues do. Bringing the subject up, no matter to whom, is the hardest part of the consultation; once this is over with, everything tends to go well. The doctor and patient create a climate of trust and

TOO MANY SUFFER IN SILENCE

One of the reasons men rarely consult doctors for sexual disorders is that they believe they are the only ones experiencing this kind of problem. It is important to remember, however, that 52% of men between the ages of 40 and 70 suffer from erectile dysfunction, and that premature ejaculation affects 35% of all men.

Men who choose not to see a doctor may hope that, in time, the problem will go away by itself. This, of course, is not always the case. They may also think that there is no effective treatment.

These preconceived ideas are stopping them from regaining their sexual health and general well-being. Only 15% of men with erectile dysfunction see their doctors. The introduction of sildenafil (Viagra) may have helped break down some important barriers, but, sadly, 85% of men still suffer in silence.

Health professionals can help. They can advise, provide information on the causes of erectile dysfunction and other sexual disorders, and suggest possible treatments.

understanding where sexual dysfunction can be addressed openly. Since I started practising, only one patient has chosen to stop seeing me because he was not comfortable enough discussing it. "

■ ERECTILE DYSFUNCTION SELF-ASSESSMENT TEST

Do you suffer from an erectile disorder? If so, does it occur rarely, occasionally or frequently? Are you worried that something is not quite normal, but still feel reluctant to speak to a doctor? A simple and quick erectile dysfunction self-assessment can help you see things more clearly and make a decision about whether to visit the doctor. The Sexual Health Inventory for Men (SHIM), developed in the United States, is one of the most widely used tests in the field. The five questions have several possible answers each, and your final score is a good indicator of the seriousness of the problem.

Circle the answer that best describes your situation:
Over the last six months...

A) *How would you rate your confidence about getting and keeping an erection?*
   1. Very low
   2. Low
   3. Moderate
   4. High
   5. Very high

B) *When your erections resulted from sexual stimulation, how often were they hard enough for penetration?*
   0. Have not been sexually activity
   1. Almost never or never
   2. A few times (much less than half the time)
   3. Sometimes (about half the time)
   4. Most times (much more than half the time)
   5. Almost always or always

C)   *During sexual intercourse, how often were you able to maintain your erection after penetrating (entering) your partner?*
  0. Did not attempt intercourse
  1. Almost never or never
  2. A few times (much less than half the time)
  3. Sometimes (about half the time)
  4. Most times (much more than half the time)
  5. Almost always or always

D)   *During sexual intercourse, how difficult was it to maintain your erection through completion of intercourse?*
  0. Did not attempt intercourse
  1. Extremely difficult
  2. Very difficult
  3. Difficult
  4. Slightly difficult
  5. Not difficult

E)   *When you attempted intercourse, how often was it satisfactory for you?*
  0. Did not attempt intercourse
  1. Almost never or never
  2. A few times (much less than half the time)
  3. Sometimes (about half the time)
  4. Most times (much more than half the time)
  5. Almost always or always

Add up the numbers you have circled. If your score is 21 or less, you may be displaying the symptoms of erectile dysfunction. If this worries you, speak to your family doctor.

■ MEDICAL ASSESSMENT: THE KEY TO DIAGNOSIS

A sexual disorder can only be diagnosed after a thorough medical assessment. This generally consists of assessment tests focusing on the patient's sexual and psychosocial background and medical history, as well as a complete medical examination. "Most of the time, this is enough detailed information to determine the presence of physiological or psychological factors," explains Dr. Dugré.

The sexual background assessment questionnaire helps the doctor discover how the sexual disorder developed. Has it always existed? If not, in what context did it first arise? Is it chronic, or does it occur only rarely? If the erections are only partial, can the patient still reach orgasm? Has the man recently changed partners? Is he experiencing a diminished sex drive? Does he experience this only with his partner, or has he lost all desire for sexual intimacy? How does the partner feel about it? Is the couple still sexually active?

The psychosocial assessment helps identify personal or relationship problems. Is the patient going through a difficult period? Has he recently lost his job or a loved one, or had any serious financial problems? Does he feel tired and depressed? Is he generally satisfied with his life? Was he a victim of sexual abuse as a child? What kind of sex education did he receive? Does he still love his partner? How is the relationship in general? Are serious disagreements (fights about the children, for example) creating a rift between the partners?

"If the man has a diminished sex drive or erectile dysfunction and the doctor suspects that he is suffering from depression, the patient may be asked to fill out the Beck Depression Inventory. If depression is detected, this assessment tool will also determine its severity. Containing a series of twenty-one questions addressing different symptoms of depression (such as sadness, work behaviour, and sexual appetite), it can be filled out at the doctor's office or at home. It is very effective and widely used by doctors."

The patient's medical history highlights any physical problems that could cause or contribute to a sexual disorder. Did the problem begin after the patient started a new medication? Does he have any other health problems? Is he suffering from a cardiovascular disease like high blood pressure or hypercholesterolemia? Does he have heart disease, diabetes or a neurological disorder? Does he smoke, drink or take drugs? Has he undergone lower abdominal or prostate surgery?

During the physical examination, the doctor will look at the cardiovascular system, secondary sex characteristics, genitalia and neurological system. This will determine whether any physical problem is contributing to the sexual disorder.

In the cardiovascular exam, blood pressure and heart rate are measured, and blood vessels in the lower limbs are palpated to check for insufficient blood flow. The doctor will also look for oedema (swelling), which in some cases is a symptom of heart failure.

Secondary sex characteristics are examined to determine whether there is atrophy or softening of the testicles. To determine whether or not a hormonal imbalance is contributing to a decrease in sex drive, the doctor also assesses the distribution of body hair and the presence or absence of abdominal obesity and gynecomasty (abnormal growth of mammary glands in males).

THE MOST IMPORTANT QUESTION
Does the patient have firm erections when he masturbates, sees erotic pictures or films, or wakes up in the morning? (Contrary to popular belief, morning erections do not result from a need to urinate).

If the answer is yes, this means the "plumbing" is working fine and the focus should shift to psychological factors.

If doctors had only five minutes to evaluate the situation, this is the question they would ask. Even though an examination and in-depth assessment are necessary to find the cause of erectile disorders, establishing the state of the basic physical mechanism is an essential preliminary.

A complete genital exam allows the doctor to detect any malformations or penile fibrosis that may indicate the existence of Peyronie's disease. A rectal exam, recommended for all men over 40, helps rule out any prostate problems that may be either linked to cancer or contributing to an ejaculation disorder.

A neurological exam is useful in cases of erectile dysfunction due to spinal injuries, multiple sclerosis or complications from diabetes. For diabetics, the test involves assessing sensitivity to vibration in the feet (patients with serious complications are unable to feel it). In other patients, the test will evaluate the strength and coordination of the lower limbs. This type of examination is sometimes necessary in cases of ejaculation disorders.

In cases of erectile dysfunction, the doctor may request a blood analysis if one has not been done in the last twelve months. Although there are unlikely to have been any changes, the test will rule out diseases like diabetes or dyslipidimea (abnormally high cholesterol levels). If the patient has less sexual desire for no apparent reason, or if the loss of desire accompanies erectile dysfunction, the doctor may request a hormonal balance test (performed on a blood sample) to check levels of testosterone, prolactin and thyroid hormones, all of which can have an impact on libido.

■ SPECIALIZED TESTS

The doctor will occasionally order further, more specialized examinations for men with erectile dysfunction to establish whether any physical disorders relating directly to the penis could be the source of the problem.

As Dr. Dugré points out, however: "These tests are not often administered because, in the past, they were ordered with a view to performing surgery on the penis (for revascularisation, for example). Today, thanks to new treatments like sildenafil (Viagra), operations are rarely necessary, which is a good thing because they can only be done in specialized institutions at a prohibitive cost that is not covered by medical insurance."

The Doppler is an ultrasound apparatus that registers blood pressure in the penis. The doctor compares it to the blood pressure in the left arm (this is called the "penobrachial index"). If the difference is too pronounced, there may be less blood flow to the arteries of the penis, which can indicate that the patient is suffering from a generalized cardiovascular disease. The Doppler Duplex is more specialized and can directly measure blood flow to the penis. These tests are simple, painless, and can be performed in twenty minutes. They may be followed up by an intracavernous injection, which causes slight discomfort. In this procedure, the doctor injects a substance into the penis that dilates the arteries and causes an erection, making assessment of the arteries and veins of the penis easier.

A nocturnal penile plethysmography is an instrument that records nocturnal erections. It measures the duration of the erections, the increase in circumference of the penis, and firmness. It is a portable instrument consisting of two rings – one placed at the base of the penis, the other at the tip – that are connected to the recording and measuring apparatus. The patient can bring it home, put it on himself and wear it for two to three consecutive nights.

If the plethysmography records no erections, or only partial ones, the erectile dysfunction probably has a physical root. If the results are normal, psychological issues should be examined as the probable cause.

After the assessment, the doctor may refer the patient to a clinic specializing in sexual disorders (a few of which can be found in Canada), or to another specialist (for example, a urologist, endocrinologist, cardiologist, neurologist or psychiatrist). Note that men with Peyronie's disease must bring a photograph of their erect penis to their urologist so the doctor can evaluate the extent of the deformation.

A sex therapist may also be called in as reinforcement to help the patient and couple explore the psychological aspects of the sexual disorder, identify possible solutions, and regain a satisfying sex life.

Even if the disorder is primarily physical, the man's psychological reaction can aggravate the problem. Occasionally, the doctor and sex therapist work in tandem, especially when the couple is in the process of integrating a new medical treatment into their life (*see chapter 7*).

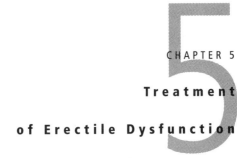

CHAPTER 5

Treatment

of Erectile Dysfunction

Dr. MICHAEL McCORMACK
Dr. LUC VALIQUETTE

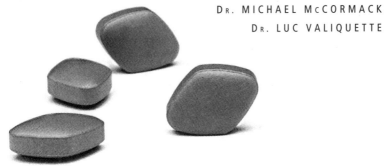

■ TREATMENTS ARE AVAILABLE

Good news! In most cases, erectile dysfunction can be successfully treated and a satisfying sex life restored. Successful treatment begins with an accurate diagnosis, which can be achieved with the help of a complete assessment, a careful physical examination and laboratory tests. Once the risk factors and the possible causes have been identified, the doctor and patient will focus on any affecting elements that might be reversed, changed, or better managed (such as smoking, diabetes, obesity, or drug prescriptions, for example). The medical treatment that follows will be chosen based on the needs and goals of both the patient and the couple. Frequently, the patient and his partner will be referred to a sex therapist.

■ SILDENAFIL (VIAGRA)

First available in 1998, Viagra was an overnight success, taking over 98% of the world market for erectile dysfunction treatments. The statistics are astounding: in the first three years, more than 20 million men world-wide were treated with Viagra. Its popularity is not difficult to understand. It is the first effective oral treatment that is easy to use, not addictive, can be taken as needed, and has very few side effects. Moreover, it works extremely well: nearly 80% of men who take it, including those with spinal injuries, have favourable results. In the very few cases that Viagra does not work, the blood vessels of the penis are so severely or completely blocked that they cannot fill with blood.

A SURPRISE DISCOVERY!
Scientists discovered the positive effects of sildenafil (Viagra) on erectile function completely by accident. In the early 1990s, the pharmaceutical company Pfizer undertook clinical trials on a new molecule targeted for the treatment of angina pectoris.

The results were rather disappointing and the researchers wanted to cancel the study. The male volunteers involved in the trial, however, wanted to continue taking the drugs... and it quickly became clear why! It turned out that they had been having excellent erections and had made the connection with the drug. Viagra was born!

An interesting bit of trivia is that the drug was named by a computer. Pharmaceutical companies often ask a computer program to make a list of words that do not exist in any language, which they then use to name their new medications. So, contrary to certain media reports at the time of its release, the name "Viagra" is not a combination of the words "vigour" and "Niagara" but simply a random computer generation.

"The success rate is even higher for men whose ED is primarily psychological: men with performance anxiety, for example, have a success rate of 90%. Viagra is less successful, however, for men with diabetes (60%) or those who have undergone a radical prostatectomy (45%). Both the disease and the operation cause severe damage to the neurological and vascular mechanisms," explains Dr. Valiquette.

HOW DOES VIAGRA WORK?
Sildenafil does not act on the brain and it does not cause erections. It simply helps men achieve and maintain erections. During sexual stimulation, the nerves of the penis emit a certain neurotransmitter that causes the blood vessels of the penis to dilate. The neuro-transmitter – cyclic GMP – is usually quickly broken down by the body, which must then produce more in order to maintain the erection. Sildenafil prevents the breakdown of cyclic GMP, making it easier to sustain erection.

Sildenafil simply gives the man a hand (so to speak) in the normal erection process. "A man who takes a Viagra pill and passively waits for an erection will be waiting for quite a while! Sildenafil cannot act on cyclic GMP without sexual stimulation."

Viagra is not, therefore, an aphrodisiac, and the man must be sexually stimulated to experience its benefits. In order to be effective, furthermore, the treatment also requires the man to change certain habits. For example, the pill has to be taken at least thirty minutes (ideally an hour) before sexual relations, which means the couple has to plan their amorous encounters a little more carefully. If the man takes the pill after a rich dinner with wine, he will have to wait one to two hours before the drug takes effect, since fatty foods and alcohol delay absorption.

"The effects of Viagra last an average of four hours. This does not mean the man has an erection for the entire time, but that he has a four-hour 'window of opportunity' to have sex, during which he can make love a few different times, if he chooses. For some men, the effects last until the following morning. It takes about 24 hours for the medication to work its way out of the system, and in order to avoid an accumulation of the drug in the body, it is necessary to wait a full day before taking another pill."

Sildenafil comes in three doses: 25 mg, 50 mg and 100 mg. The dosage prescribed will depend on the man's general health, the seriousness of the erectile problem and the possible interactions with other medications he might be taking. The doctor will decide which dosage is appropriate. "The man should not take two or three pills at once, or take it more often in the hopes of increasing its effectiveness. This simply doesn't work. Once maximum effectiveness has been reached, any extra amounts of medication

IS SILDENAFIL (VIAGRA ™ *) A SAFE WAY TO TREAT ED?
Yes, unless:

- the man is currently taking or is going to take nitro-glycerine or another nitrate-based medication. When combined with Viagra, these substances can cause a sharp drop in blood pressure which, depending on the state of the patient's heart, can be fatal.
- the man is suffering from symptoms of high blood pressure.
- the man has chest pain during sexual relations.
- the man has recently suffered a heart attack or a stroke.
- the man is taking "poppers" (a type of recreational drug) or "Spanish Fly" (an "aphrodisiac" sold in sex paraphernalia shops). These substances are nitrate derivatives and they can also cause a drop in blood pressure.

Consult your physician if you have questions.

* Pfizer Products Inc., Pfizer Canada Inc., licence holder.

will only add to the side effects. It should be noted, however, that an overdose of Viagra is not really dangerous."

SIDE EFFECTS AND CONTRAINDICATIONS

The most common side effects of Viagra are headaches, facial flushing, upset stomach and nasal congestion. "In most patients, the effects are benign, easily tolerated and temporary. However, it is always wise to tell your doctor or pharmacist about any effects you may be experiencing, and it is never a good idea to share your medication with another person. Some men are allergic to various ingredients in Viagra, although this is rare." One interesting side effect is seeing the world through blue-tinted glasses! In about 3% of users, the drug acts on an enzyme that distinguishes colours. In these cases, men's vision is slightly tinged with blue for the first four hours after they have taken the drug, but this is not dangerous at all and in no way affects their vision.

For most men, sildenafil is harmless, even if they have heart disease. "If the cardiologist or the family doctor confirms that the patient's heart is strong enough for him to have sexual relations, he can take Viagra – on condition, of course, that he is not taking any nitrates or nitrate derivatives. If there is any doubt, always ask the doctor or cardiologist."

There is no need for concern about whether Viagra carries a risk of heart attack. Pfizer has performed rigorous scientific studies

SIDE EFFECTS

Headache:	16%
Facial flushing:	10%
Digestion problems:	6.5%
Bluish vision:	3%
Nasal congestion:	4.2%
Diarrhea:	2%
Dizziness:	2%

involving thousands of men, and none of this research has established a link between sildenafil and heart attack.

Viagra has helped a great many men deal with erectile dysfunction. It is not, however, a magic drug; it cannot resolve discord in a relationship, or bring back sexual desire. These problems require the help of a sex therapist, who may also help if a man or his partner is having trouble adapting to Viagra because it makes their sex life seem too artificial.

It should also be remembered that this product does not work for all men. Six to eight unsuccessful tries indicate that it is not effective for a particular user. There are, however other efficacious treatments.

▩ OTHER SOLUTIONS

TRANSURETHRAL TREATMENT (MUSE)

The Medicated Urethral System of Erection (MUSE) consists of inserting a mini-suppository of alprostadil, the size of a grain of rice (1.4 mm wide by 3 to 6 mm long, depending on the concentration), into the urethra. The medication is absorbed through the urethral walls and carried by the blood to the cavernous bodies of the penis, where it acts in the same way as injected alprostadil. The product does not, however, absorb as effectively this way as it does through intracavernous injections, and is successful in only about 40% of cases.

The technique is performed as follows: after urinating, the mini-suppository is inserted into the opening at the end of the penis (the urinary meatus) with an applicator. The penis must then be lightly massaged to accelerate absorption and increase effectiveness. The erection occurs within 20 minutes (sexual stimulation is not necessary) and generally lasts under an hour, whether or not there is ejaculation. During this time, the penis will remain erect even if sexual relations come to an end.

"MUSE is contraindicated for any man who has a blood disorder that predisposes him to priapism. This drug has very few undesirable side effects other than an occasional burning sensation during urination and unpleasant feeling in the urethra (in 36% of cases), the latter most frequently a problem for diabetics. If the man's partner is pregnant, he must wear a condom, since the drug can cause contractions in the uterus. Furthermore, the effects of the medication on a foetus are unknown, so it is recommended that the couple use some form of birth control if there is a chance the woman may become pregnant. If the couple is actually trying to conceive, the man should not use the MUSE method," emphasizes Dr. McCormack.

MUSE® – TRANSURETHRAL TREATMENT *

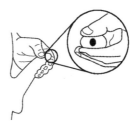

Either sitting or standing, gently extend the penis upwards as far as possible, exerting light pressure from the tip to the base. This will straighten and open the urethra.

Slowly insert the applicator into the urethra. Be sure to insert the applicator as far as the projecting rim, in order to ensure absorption of the medicated pellet.

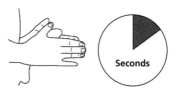

Hold the penis in an upward position, extending it as far as possible. Firmly roll the penis between the hands for at least 10 seconds to ensure that the medication is distributed along the walls of the urethra.

Seconds

Get up and walk around for 10 minutes while the erection appears. Physical activity increases blood flow to the penis and improves the quality of the erection. Wait at least 10 minutes more before beginning sexual relations.

Minutes

MUSE is a registered trademark of Vivus Pharmaceuticals.

INTRACAVERNOUS (PENILE) INJECTIONS

This treatment has been used since the early 1980s, and is effective in more than 85% of cases, whatever the cause of the erectile dysfunction. However, because the idea of administering an injection directly to the penis is generally unpleasant to men, half of those prescribed this method quickly abandon it, while others simply reject it outright, mistakenly believing it to be painful or dangerous.

The treatment requires that the man inject a drug, or a combination of drugs, into the side of the penis, directly into one of the cavernous bodies (the two are interconnected). The substances used are alprostadil (known on the market as Caverject®), papaverine (an opium derivative), phentolamine, or a mixture of the three. These drugs cause the muscles of the arterial walls and cavernous bodies to relax, allowing the organ to become engorged with blood. Within fifteen minutes, even without sexual stimulation, the penis will become completely firm and the erection will last for an average of thirty minutes to an hour. It may persist for some time even after ejaculation and the termination of sexual activity.

"The doctor must show the patient how to administer the injection so he won't cause ecchymosis (benign bleeding beneath the skin of the penis). The first few times, the injection may bring on a slight cramp in the man's penis. A few attempts are necessary to determine the appropriate dose for the patient," says Dr. McCormack. "It is also

INTRACAVERNOUS INJECTION

Injectable area
(shaded)

Cross-section of penis
showing correct needle
position in the cavernous
body

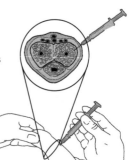

recommended that the man choose a different spot to inject as often as he can in order to avoid scarring, which could potentially cause a deformation of the penis similar to that of Peyronie's disease." Furthermore, injections should not be administered more than once every 24 hours, since an overdose can lead to priapism.

This treatment is contraindicated in exceptional cases where the man is allergic to one of the products, or has a blood disorder that predisposes him to priapism. Patients taking anticoagulant drugs (to thin the blood) must also be very careful not to cause a haemorrhage or hematoma when injecting the medication. Men with a phobia of needles are not advised to use this treatment. It is also not recommended for those who have vision problems (they must be able to see well to properly administer the injection), trembling hands (from Parkinson's disease, for example), or a problem with obesity (if this obscures their view of the penis). Diabetics, already accustomed to using a syringe for insulin injections, are generally the best candidates for this technique.

QUITE A DOCTOR!
The first proof that intracavernous injections were an effective treatment was presented to the medical community in a rather unique manner.

No one had ever believed that drugs injected into the cavernous bodies of the penis could actually produce a quick and reliable erection. Then, in 1983, during an American Urological Association conference in Las Vegas, British scientist Dr. Giles Brindley provided some indisputable proof to the contrary.

Dr. Brindley injected the product into his own penis, and with his pants down, walked around the room, to the stupefaction and uproarious laughter of the audience. Now that's solid evidence!

The most important thing to watch out for is the duration of the erection. If it persists for more than four hours, there is a strong risk of priapism (which can occasionally occur, especially when using papaverine). In such a case, the man must go to an emergency room where he will be given an antidote to suppress the erection.

VACUUM PUMP
This mechanism is an external prosthesis – a cylinder open at one end that is connected by a tube to a vacuum pump. The penis is inserted into the hermetically sealed cylinder, and a vacuum is created by the pump which draws the blood into the penis. A security valve allows the man to control the pressure, so it does

VACUUM PUMP

After the penis is inserted into the cylinder, the pump creates a vacuum drawing blood into the penis.

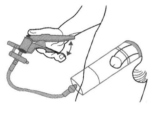

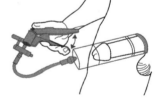

Within minutes, the vacuum causes an erection.

Slide the ring sealing the cylinder to the base of the penis, and withdraw the cylinder.

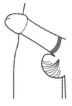

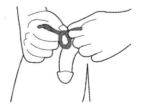

Once the ring is removed from the penis, the organ will return to its normal flaccid state.

no damage to the tissues. The pump brings the penis to firmness within a few minutes, without sexual stimulation. Once the erection has been achieved, an elastic ring is placed around the base of the penis to sustain it. The cylinder and pump are then removed, and sexual relations can take place.

The compression ring cannot be left in place for more than 30 to 45 minutes. If left on longer, the cells in the penis are deprived of oxygen and there is a risk of blood clotting, which can cause permanent damage to the inside of the cavernous bodies. Many men do not like the feeling of the ring and find it uncomfortable; nor do they like the fact that their penis becomes cold because of the temporary loss of circulation. The effect is like that of placing an elastic band tightly around the base of a finger.

"The mechanical nature of this method is a turn-off for many men," says Dr. McCormack. "It takes practice to learn how to use it, but once mastered, the man can get an erection in moments. Couples who have become used to this technique say that it works about 80% of the time. There is only one contraindication: men taking anticoagulants, such as coumadin for heart disease, thrombophlebitis, or as a treatment for stroke or other disorders, should not use this method. Because this drug stops the blood from coagulating, any small injury to the penis caused by the prosthesis or ring may cause the penis to lose blood (causing a hematoma or bruise). One piece of advice: don't skimp when purchasing the pump or the compression ring. The quality of the mechanism can make all the difference between failure and success."

PENILE IMPLANTS

The practice of inserting penile implants or "supports" into the two cavernous bodies of the penis has existed since the early 1970s and is effective in the vast majority of cases. Very rarely, the implants must be removed because of infection. There are two models: semi-rigid (malleable) and inflatable.

The semi-rigid prosthesis is made of a metal rod covered by silicone, one of which is inserted into each cavernous body. There are several advantages to this type of prosthesis: it is less expensive than the inflatable models, less mechanically complicated, rarely breaks, and is relatively easy to insert. With this model, the penis is always "ready to go," since it is in a permanent state of semi-erection firm enough for penetration. For this very reason, however, it is also more difficult to conceal, even though newer models have more malleable metal rods.

The form and function of the inflatable prosthesis imitate a normal penis. It is made of two cylinders, a reservoir of saline water and a hydraulic pump. The cylinders are inserted into the cavernous bodies of the penis and the reservoir implanted in the abdomen. Everything is connected to a pump, which has been inserted into the scrotum. When the patient activates the pump (by pressing and releasing the inflation button hidden in the scrotum), the saline water enters the cylinders and inflates the cavernous bodies to complete erection. Once sexual relations are finished, the man presses on the pump valve to send the liquid back to the reservoir, and the penis becomes flaccid. Compared to the semi-rigid prosthesis, this model is much more expensive, more complicated to implant, and more likely to run into mechanical failures that will necessitate surgery again.

Even though the technique has been refined over the years, prosthesis implantation is still an irreversible surgery and carries with it potential risks and complications. The most common concerns are infections of the prosthesis (in which case the mechanism must be removed), and malfunctions of the mechanism due to faulty adjustment or a mechanical problem. The implantation of the prosthesis also causes an irreversible fibrosis in the cavernous bodies of the penis, permanently destroying the natural erectile mechanism. Therefore, if the prothesis must be removed and another one cannot be reimplanted, the man will never be able to have an erection again. While penile implants are a possibility for diabetics, they run a greater risk of infection.

In the past, penile implants were the primary treatment for men with erectile problems. Because much less invasive methods have now been developed, however, the technique is used only as a last resort. Because of the irreversible consequences of the procedure, it is recommended only if all other methods have failed.

ALTERNATIVE METHODS

Some men try to resolve their erectile dysfunction problems with so-called "natural" products because it makes them feel they have more control over their bodies, because they do not like taking drugs, or simply because they feel they have nothing to lose and think these treatments are safe.

Modern Western medicine does not necessarily have all the answers. Some unknown or little-known natural substances that have beneficial effects on sexual function certainly exist. However, scientific knowledge about many dietary supplements is limited because there has been very little serious study of these products.

Why have there been so few scientific studies of natural products? "For the very simple reason that the companies that make these products have nothing to gain by undertaking them!" says Dr. McCormack. "If a producer submits a product to rigorous scientific trials, following all the rules, the product will be moved to the official category of a drug and therefore become subject to strict and costly regulations. Furthermore, the study may prove that the product is not effective. Generally, they have a lot more to gain by simply letting word of mouth give their products a reputation."

Anabolic steroids are very popular with body-builders because they increase body mass and muscular strength, creating a kind of "superman." It is therefore not surprising that some men suffering from erectile dysfunction are interested in taking these drugs. Those most commonly used for this purpose are androstenedione and dehydroepiandrosterone (better known as DHEA). They are not legal in Canada

It is thought that these two substances, composed of natural products, are transformed into testosterone (among other things) by the male body, and that this can have an effect on the libido. However, no studies have confirmed this. Furthermore, three trials have shown that androstenedione may have negative effects on a man's general health (by reducing the levels of HDL, or "good" cholesterol) and even his cardiovascular health (although this has yet to be confirmed). As for DHEA, the pills containing the substance usually have such a low dosage that there is no effect whatsoever on erectile capacity. Moreover, no research has shown any beneficial effects of this drug for men suffering from sexual dysfunction.

Gingko biloba is an extract from the leaves of a tree native to Asia. It is said to have beneficial effects on degenerative diseases (such as Alzheimer's), and may be able to slow the aging process and help men achieve erection. "Here, again, no scientific studies have proven

REAL OR PLACEBO EFFECT?

The question of whether alternative or so-called "natural" products have a real effect or simply act as placebos deserves a closer look.

When the researchers of a pharmaceutical company study a drug, they separate the volunteers into two groups: one takes the drug, the other a placebo (a substance that contains no medication). The subjects of the study do not know who has been given what. In studies on erectile dysfunction treatments, it was found that 25% of the men who took the placebo said their erections had improved. The effect, of course, was entirely psychological.

This 25% is important when considering the claims of effectiveness by producers of "natural" products. If they proudly announce that their product is effective 25% to 30% of the time, we can deduce that their product is no more effective than a placebo, which throws the genuine efficacy of the product into question.

The best thing to do is speak to a doctor.

its effectiveness as a treatment for erectile dysfunction. However, it has been shown that it acts as an anticoagulant. Therefore, anyone taking anticoagulant drugs like aspirin or coumadin must not take gingko because the combination of the two can cause internal bleeding."

Yohimbine is an extract from the bark the yohimbe tree, which grows in Africa. In the past, some doctors prescribed it for erectile dysfunction, although this is no longer the case, since it has been proven to be ineffective. Furthermore, yohimbine has certain negative side effects, such as palpitations, flushing, high blood pressure, insomnia and panic attacks.

L-arginine, an essential amino acid, is one of the so-called "natural" products that is of interest to scientists. "L-arginine has a number of effects, including the production of neurotransmitter chemicals that are necessary for erection. Two serious studies have concluded that men who lacked these neurotransmitters benefited from taking L-arginine supplements. While it has not yet been shown to be effective for all men with erectile dysfunction, the molecule is promising and scientists are in the process of trying to create an effective drug from it. The supplements are available on Internet Web sites (they are not available in Canada), but do not have concentrations strong enough to improve erection." This amino acid is also found in food, particularly in vegetables, whole grains and nuts. It is sometimes said that eating five grams of nuts a day can help a man with his erections, and it may be true. At any rate, there is no harm in trying!

"There are also other products that claim to have aphrodisiac qualities, such as ginseng, avena sativa, tribulus terrestris and turnera diffusa. The effectiveness of these dietary supplements is unclear, and only scientific research can help us determine whether or not they are useful. The same can be said about 'soft' medicine, like acupuncture, reflexology or homeopathy. We are not saying they are ineffective; we are simply emphasizing that their effectiveness has not been scientifically proven," concludes Dr. McCormack.

WHAT WILL THE FUTURE BRING?

The appearance of sildenafil (Viagra) has profoundly changed the therapeutic approach to erectile dysfunction. The eager acceptance shown by patients and the drug's proven effectiveness has pushed researchers to find comparable products, or new uses for existing products. Three other oral medications, tadalafil, vardenafil and apomorphine, will probably find their way to the Canadian market in the near future.

Tadalafil and vardenafil belong to the same therapeutic class as sildenafil. This means they act in the same way and have more or less the same side effects. It is too early to make comparisons between these products, but more information will be available soon. Apomorphine is different from the others because of its mechanism of action. It acts on the central nervous system, stimulating brain impulses (nerve messages) to the penis. Nausea is the primary side effect. It does not interact with nitrate derivatives so patients taking nitrate-based medications will probably be able to use it.

The future may also bring other methods of administering sildenafil (Viagra), such as a nasal vaporizer or sublingual patch that melts under the tongue. Researchers are also studying the feasibility of administering alprostadil (the substance contained in MUSE and Caverject) in gel or cream form, or with skin patches. Phentolamine, a substance already used in intracavernous injections, may also become available in oral preparations.

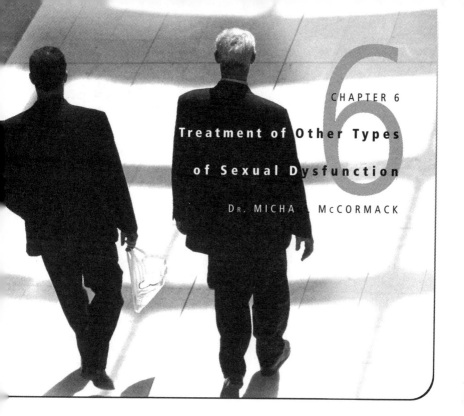

▦ PREMATURE EJACULATION

It should be mentioned, by way of introduction, that the incidence of premature ejaculation tends to decrease with age. Although it does not disappear altogether, the majority of older men are better at restraining themselves from orgasm. "It is difficult to say exactly why this is so. It may be because the skin of the penis becomes less sensitive with age," says Dr. McCormack. "Whatever the reason, men do not have to wait until they are fifty to fix the problem. We can help them long before that!"

Antidepressants are often prescribed as treatment for premature ejaculation, not because the man has a psychological problem, but because they act on the nervous system to retard the ejaculatory reflex. For the first three weeks of treatment, the patient takes one pill a day. After that, the dosage decreases to one pill two or three hours before sexual relations, as long as the man can predict it.

The antidepressant does not have any significant effect on mood or erectile function since the patient takes lower and fewer doses than those taking the drug for depression. Although this treatment is effective in 70% of cases, many men still resist it because of the psychological connotations, as well as the need to predict lovemaking in advance.

Another treatment is intracavernous injections, which are also used to treat erectile dysfunction (*see chapter 5*). "The erection lasts an average of an hour and continues after ejaculation. The man still reaches orgasm quickly, but can now at least sustain his erection long enough to satisfy his partner." Injections can be taken as needed or as desired; unless he wants to, it is not essential that a man use it every time he makes love. This treatment can also be taken temporarily to help men suffering from performance anxiety recover their confidence.

Perineal re-education, or the strengthening of the pelvic floor muscles, may also be suggested. Kegel exercises (the same as those recommended for new mothers) can help the man delay ejaculation. The exercises are very simple: contract the buttocks and anus for ten seconds and repeat for fifteen minutes, two or three times a day. Performing this exercise while making love is an easy trick and can be very effective in delaying ejaculation.

Penis sensitivity can be decreased with specially designed anaesthetic creams, sold over the counter. "The substance numbs the skin, a little like the topical ointment used by dentists. The man applies it to the glans (the head of the penis), puts on a condom to ensure the cream is absorbed, and after thirty minutes (the time required for the product to fully penetrate), is ready to make love, keeping the condom on so the vagina doesn't also become desensitized. It is a simple, inexpensive solution for those who don't like taking drugs, and is effective in about 40% of cases." There are some problems with this technique, however. Keeping the condom on for thirty minutes can sometimes be problematic, and because the cream numbs the skin of the penis, it diminishes the man's pleasure and makes it more difficult for him to sustain erection.

"Some men who suffer from premature ejaculation wear a condom (or perhaps more than one) during sex, which reduces their level of excitement and delays orgasm. But this doesn't work for everyone. Some men prefer to masturbate or be masturbated by their partner so they can have a 'quickie' orgasm first and last longer the 'second time around.' Other men can better control their orgasm by increasing the frequency of their sexual contact. Making love only once a month certainly makes it harder to hold back!"

Since there are no contraindications for any of these methods, the man is free to try all of them before choosing the one that suits him best.

Sex therapy is another option. Results are excellent, with success rates of up to 95%, even when the premature ejaculation has a physical origin, such as hypersensitivity of the skin of the penis. The sex therapist can help the man "tame" his sexual excitement. Combining sex therapy and medical treatment maximizes the man's chances of success (*see chapter 7*).

■ DELAYED EJACULATION AND ANEJACULATION

Unfortunately, there are no effective medical treatments for delayed ejaculation or anejaculation. "Other than changing a medication that has brought the condition on, the doctor really has no solution. Since it is believed that there is often a psychological component to the disorder, sex therapy may be an option. If this does not help, the only thing the patient can do is learn to live with the problem."

"However," Dr. McCormack continues, "this sexual dysfunction is rare, and most men dealing with it usually do just fine. Once they have been reassured that it does not pose a danger to their health, it doesn't seem to bother them much."

What if they want to start a family? "They usually manage to do it the natural way. Delayed ejaculation or anejaculation does not actually mean that the man never ejaculates. In most cases, 'normal' sex does happen occasionally (once every five, ten or twenty times, for example)." In the worst cases, the couple may resort to medically assisted reproduction techniques.

If a sex therapist is involved, he or she will try to determine the underlying cause of the problem and suggest exercises to help the man learn to relax, let himself go and appreciate sexual contact.

■ RETROGRADE EJACULATION

If a drug is the cause of the problem, the doctor will modify the prescription. If not, retrograde ejaculation is, at least in principle, an irreversible problem.

"Before performing a transurethral prostatectomy for benign hypertrophy of the prostate, the surgeon warns the patient that the surgery will affect the mechanism coordinating the closure between the bladder and urethra and cause retrograde ejaculation. Because this usually affects men over the age of fifty who generally no longer intend to start a family, the fact that their sperm is re-directed to the bladder rather than being expelled out the penis does not really bother them."

However, the situation is different for a young man who has undergone pelvic surgery (such as surgery for testicular cancer). When he is ready to start a family, the doctor can prescribe a medication known as an alphastimulant, which temporarily closes the bladder neck. The patient should take it as long as it takes for the couple to conceive, but doctors do not recommend it for long-term use as it causes heart palpitations.

These medical problems do not usually require the intervention of a sex therapist.

■ PEYRONIE'S DISEASE

The doctor must wait twelve to eighteen months, until the disease is through the progressive stage, before intervening. Many men, however, are too worried to wait that long and try to find another way to stop the deformation process. Various "miracle" cures, in the form of ultrasound mechanisms, pills or ointments, are available on the Internet or in magazine ads, but none are effective.

"One of the potential solutions is vitamin E. As an antioxidant, it can help preserve some of the elasticity of the penis and control the extent of the deformation. It is recommended that patients take 400 IU (international units) a day (there is no need to consult a doctor). Vitamin E creams for direct application to the penis are not recommended because the cream doesn't absorb as well as the pills; nor can using the cream at the same time as taking the pills in any way increase the chances of improvement."

Once the acute period of the disease has passed, the doctor and patient discuss the options and come to a decision based on what would most improve the patient's quality of life. If the penis has basically returned to its normal state and sexual relations are going reasonably well, the patient will probably not choose surgery; if the curvature is quite pronounced, however, he likely will. "The operation straightens the penis. It is not major surgery (the patient can go home after 24 hours) and it is less painful than one might think thanks to highly effective modern anaesthetic methods. The man will be able to make love four weeks later."

It should be noted that the operation will shorten the penis by one or two centimetres, an inevitable consequence of straightening it. Of course, the patient is made aware of this before deciding whether or not to have surgery. "Most men decide that it's worth it when the alternative is to not be able to make love at all." In addition to the shortening, the patient should also be aware that the surgeon will circumcise him to accelerate the healing of the skin.

"The operation merely straightens the penis; the fibrous plaque is not removed. Although this can be done with surgery, the procedure is very risky and does not really lead to better results. Therefore, if the fibrosis has made the man's penis soft at the tip (above the fibrosis) it will stay that way." After the operation, these cases must be treated like other erectile problems, with sildenafil (Viagra). There is no need to worry, however. Even if the fibrous plaque remains, there is no danger that the disease will come back.

A sex therapist can help the man accept the changes to his body, as well as understand that he can continue to have a satisfying sex life.

PRIAPISM

As noted in chapter 3, priapism is a dangerous condition. If the man's erection has lasted for more than four hours, he should go directly to the emergency room. First, the doctor will try to suppress the erection by pumping the blood out of the penis with a needle. If that doesn't work, an antidote (adrenaline or epinephrine) will be injected to contract the muscles of the penis, causing the blood to drain back into the body. In almost every case, the erection disappears immediately. If it does not, an emergency operation can drain the blood.

The patient may be kept for 24 hours for observation, but he is generally sent home immediately. The doctor will probably require a follow-up visit after a few weeks to ensure that everything is in order. There is no need for psychological intervention.

If the patient waits more than four hours to consult, the accumulation of blood in the penis may cause the formation of a clot that will be impossible to dissolve. The doctor will be able to suppress the erection, but the damage to the tissues of the penis might be irreversible. The man will never be able to have normal erections again, and the only help available to him would be penile implants.

LOWERED SEX DRIVE

If the man's loss of desire can be explained by a health problem (anemia, diabetes, hypogonadism, etc.), the doctor will prescribe medications to treat the disease. If the problem is the result of alcohol or drug consumption, the patient can be helped to overcome his addiction. If a medication is responsible, the doctor can change the prescription.

"However, in cases where psychological elements are primary, the best the doctor can do is refer the patient to a sex therapist," says Dr. McCormack.

The sex therapist's evaluation will be thorough and intensive, since there are so many possible reasons for diminished desire (the arrival of a first child, conflict in the couple, sexual frustration, monotony, to name only a few). Several methods of treatment will be explored in the following chapter.

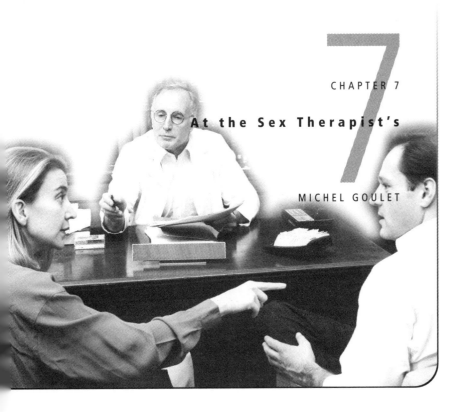

▪ WHY CONSULT A SEX THERAPIST?

Sexology is the science of sexuality and sexual disorders and was developed only thirty years ago. "Our role is to provide people with the tools and support to help them discover or recuperate a satisfying sex life. Since all aspects of the personality must be taken into account, sex therapy has a lot in common with psychotherapy," says Michel Goulet.

Although you can consult with a sex therapist directly, he or she may refer you to a medical doctor if the evaluation process reveals the possibility of a physical explanation. It is therefore better to rule out any physical causes at the beginning by going to see a medical doctor first.

A doctor will refer his or her patient to a sex therapist if there is reason to believe the sexual problem is psychological. The services of a sex therapist are not free, but the cost is covered by some insurance plans. Consulting a sex therapist may also be recommended if the doctor believes it can help the patient (and couple) overcome a physical problem or learn how to live with one (for example, in the case of a man who becomes paralysed and is no longer able to achieve an erection). A sex therapist can provide support for all kinds of sexual disorders, including erectile dysfunction, ejaculation problems, diminished sex drive, and performance anxiety.

"Even though men are generally more open these days, they can still be apprehensive about discussing their sexuality. They feel the subject is too personal, or that they will be judged. This is perfectly normal, but men should remember that the sex therapist has already heard thousands of stories and is there to help, not criticize. The longer a man hesitates, the worse the problem can become."

Some medical doctors across the country with advanced training in sexuality and sexual disorders also practice sexology. While some practice both medicine and therapy, most generally only perform medical evaluations and prescribe treatment if necessary.

HOW TO CHOOSE A SEX THERAPIST

The University of Quebec at Montreal (UQAM) has offered a sexology programme since 1975. In fact, Quebec is the only province in Canada where it is possible to get a degree in the subject.

In Quebec, only sex therapists with a master's degree specializing in counselling are qualified to practice sex therapy. Always be sure to check qualifications.

In other provinces, many psychologists and social workers provide sex therapy services. Their methods are very similar to those used in Quebec. It is recommended that you choose a psychologist or a social worker with a master's degree, since this ensures they have received training in psychotherapy.

A final question: is it better to choose a man or a woman? This is, of course, entirely up to you. And always remember that if you don't feel comfortable with the sex therapist you have chosen, you can always find a new one.

■ GO WITH YOUR PARTNER

The first meeting with the sex therapist usually lasts about one hour. The sex therapist will conduct a simple interview and perform an evaluation (questionnaires are sometimes used, especially when trying to detect depression). If the man is in a relationship, the sex therapist will usually request that his partner be present for the interview, and may take a few minutes aside with each of them. "The presence of the partner can help us learn a great deal about the quality of the relationship," explains Mr. Goulet. "The partner will undoubtedly have questions that need to be answered too, and can also usually offer a more objective account of the problem."

When did the sexual problem first occur? Is it intermittent or chronic? Can a particular event explain it? Did this problem occur with other partners? Is the relationship a happy one? Is it as happy as it has always been? Do the partners still make love and if so, how frequently? Is sex unsatisfying for both partners? Are they able to talk about it? Has it created tension between them? These are the kind of questions the sex therapist will ask in the first interview.

"The two partners will often have different answers, which is why the man's partner should participate in the sharing of information; the more complete the data, the more successful the therapy is likely to be. However, some men are more modest or shy than others, and may prefer to come to the first meeting alone (unless the problem has already been identified as one directly involving both partners, such as decreased desire due to conflict within the couple). This is legitimate, but we should be aware that sexual disorders have an impact on both partners, and the relationship has a better chance of survival if the couple faces the problem together."

Sexual disorders can, in fact, destroy a relationship. Erectile dysfunction or premature ejaculation, for example, can have a negative effect on a man's self-confidence. He may think to himself, "I'm no good in bed," or "Why would anyone love me?", or he could fear, "Is she going to lose interest in me?" His partner may think, "He doesn't want me anymore," or "He just wants to get it over with." She may go as far as to think, "He must be getting satisfaction somewhere else." This can create palpable tension, which can come out in hurtful sarcasm or statements like, "You never want to make love anymore," or "You're not the man you used to be."

Unfortunately, this type of reaction is common and only makes the situation worse. After a while, the man will very likely withdraw (by ceasing to communicate or display affection) and invest more time and

TIMES HAVE CHANGED!

The clientele consulting sex therapists has changed a great deal over the last 30 years.

In the 1970s, resources for sexual matters were usually fairly scarce. Sexual morality was still quite strict, and there were a lot of taboos. People who did consult sex therapists usually went because they needed information. Most questions centred on subjects like conception, techniques of giving and receiving sexual pleasure, or clearing up misconceptions regarding female or male sexuality.

These days, things are quite different. A vast amount of information is easily accessible via books, television shows, the Internet, articles, and other media. As a result, sex therapists receive fewer requests to provide educational services alone. Cases are now much more complex and require deeper analysis. This development has made the profession all the more challenging and exciting!

effort in his work to forget his problems, or isolate himself socially. Some men can fall into a major depression. The relationship can move closer and closer to a break-up without either one of the partners even realizing that a sexual disorder is at the root of their troubles.

■ SEX THERAPY

After the evaluation, the sex therapist will likely recommend sex therapy. "This is a clinical process where the sex therapist provides his or her patients and their partners with different approaches to finding a solution for their sexual problem."

And what are these approaches? There are four approaches used by the various professionals in the sexual health field: cognitive-behaviour (the most common), systemic, sexoanalysis, and humanist-existential. No one approach is better than the other, and they may all be adapted to suit different situations. It is also possible to integrate more than one approach in therapy if this promises to better serve the patient. Sex therapy is conducted in weekly sessions and can last from 15 to 30 weeks (the ideal frequency for optimal results). It is rare for a treatment to last more than a year, but this may be necessary in cases of profound psychological trauma or deep-set sexual problems.

It is interesting to note that sex therapy was introduced by the famous American researchers, Masters and Johnson. Their work was single-handedly responsible for moving the field of sexual medicine from the Stone Age into the modern era. Before sex therapy, people suffering from sexual problems usually just had to learn to live with them. The few methods that did exist (like couples' therapy) gave very poor results, as they did not examine the sexual aspect of the relationship in any depth. (Of course, it should be remembered that we now have a great deal more knowledge about human sexuality than we did then.)

Although it is often successful, sex therapy is not always recommended. If the patient is not in very good mental health –

for example, if he has major depression – this may not be the time for sex therapy. He should consult a psychiatrist or a psychologist first, and then determine if it is possible to undergo parallel treatment in sex therapy. Nor is sex therapy recommended for couples with severely damaged relationships and a deep fear of intimacy with each other. In cases like this, sexual disorders are not their main difficulties, and the sex therapist may decide to refer them to another professional.

As with the initial interview, the partner's participation throughout the therapy can contribute greatly to its success (unless, of course, the man is single and consulting the sex therapist to deal with a problem such as premature ejaculation). It is easier to resolve conflicts that can arise during therapy if the partner is involved in the treatment. It also makes it possible to verify whether one party or other is unconsciously "sabotaging" the process. This can occur in a number of ways. For example, one partner may not be fully committed to the therapy, refuse to participate out of anger, or block the process because he or she is afraid of changing the dynamics within the couple.

The partner does not need to be present at each session, but his or her involvement at some level should be encouraged, especially

CAN'T AFFORD SEX THERAPY?

What can you do if you do not have enough money to pay for sex therapy?

You can look for a clinic or a hospital in your area that offers internship positions. Interns in sexology, social work or psychology can provide very good service for free or a nominal fee.

If no interns are available, you may find a professional who is willing to accept a lower rate. Your family doctor can also help you find someone.

if the couple is experiencing communication problems. If both partners are at most or all of the sessions, they will both get the same information and have a comparable understanding of it. "What one partner brings home is not always exactly what the sex therapist said! Messages can be oddly distorted as they are relayed. I have had patients," Mr. Goulet goes on, laughing, "who went and told their partners that the sex therapist had 'prescribed' sex three times a week, when it was in fact the patients themselves who wanted to make love that often!"

■ COGNITIVE-BEHAVIOUR THERAPY

This approach focuses on any negative thoughts the person has about his sexuality that can lead to negative emotions and cause sexual problems. "An individual's perception can be constantly coloured by negativity. It is like he is wearing tinted glasses without knowing it. Simply becoming conscious of it can help him get rid of this destructive view and see things more clearly."

For example, a man suffering from erectile dysfunction because of diabetes may have come to fear making love with his wife because he is convinced he cannot satisfy her. His negative thoughts only aggravate the situation, paralysing his desire and his sexual capacity to the point where he is no longer capable of achieving satisfying erections. Cognitive-behaviour therapy tries to break this fear-born vicious circle by modifying or diminishing the power of negative thoughts. "We try to help the patient clearly identify his thoughts at the moment of sexual relations – thoughts like 'This is not going to work.' We also examine the partner's perception: maybe she is actually perfectly satisfied with his performance! The man may learn to demand less of himself and see sexuality as more than penetration alone."

"Cognitive-behaviour therapy can also be used to treat a man whose doctor wants to prescribe sildenafil (Viagra), but who refuses to take any sort of medication. He may be under the impression that taking Viagra means he is no longer a real man. Sex therapy can help him change this erroneous perception. The sex therapist can then ask the doctor to prescribe the drug (since only doctors can write prescriptions). By defusing his negative thoughts about the drug itself, the sex therapist can help the patient integrate Viagra into his sex life. In the course of the therapy, the patient can also learn about other sources of sexual pleasure (caresses, masturbation, etc.) that will allow him to take the medication less frequently or for a shorter period."

This approach can also be used when a man no longer wants to make love, but cannot understand why, since he claims to love his partner. "During therapy, we may come to see that the man has always been afraid of rejection and that over the years has become less and less self-confident. Afraid of being abandoned by his partner, he avoids all intimate behaviour that can bring him closer to what he can lose. His fear of rejection blocks his access to pleasure. Or, another man who has just started a family may feel, on an unconscious level, that now that his wife is a mother, she can no longer be his lover. He removes her from any sexual identity and associates her primarily with madonna-like virtue." In both cases, the sex therapist can help the patient readjust to reality.

"However, if it becomes clear that the decrease in desire is more clearly linked to problems such as bad communication within the couple, boredom, or difficulty managing conflict around the children, the sex therapist will apply systemic therapy," explains Mr. Goulet. He further emphasizes that lack of desire is one of the most difficult problems to treat, since it is usually extremely complex.

■ SYSTEMIC THERAPY

This approach focuses on the couple and is used when both partners appear to share equal responsibility for the problem. In other words, systemic therapy is used when the couple wants to "work on their relationship" in a way similar to that of marriage counselling.

The aim of the approach is to understand the interaction of the couple and its effects on their sex life. The sex therapist can then use certain (primarily communicative) tools to help iron out the difficulties and make the relationship less complicated and more harmonious.

For example, a 55-year-old man has remarried a younger woman of 30. She wants children. He does not, but does not dare admit it. Over time, the man may develop erectile dysfunction that is directly related to his fear of having children. The sex therapist will first try to understand the man's concerns and help clarify his position (this would require a few individual sessions). The sex therapist will then try to help him open up to his partner and express his opinion so that she can have all the information required to make a decision about the relationship.

Men with spinal cord injuries who are paralysed from the waist down can also benefit from this approach, as it can help them adapt to their new sexual reality. Although certain treatments may allow them to achieve erections again, nothing will ever be quite the same. Sex therapists can teach couples in this situation to use their senses, take pleasure in caresses, and enjoy their fantasies, among other techniques. "The most important sexual organ is the brain! The act of concentrating on other sensations and parts of the body can be extremely pleasurable. People can learn that sexuality takes different forms and can become even more satisfying.

"Systemic therapy is also helpful for the great number of men who seek help for premature ejaculation. Very often, they explain it by saying their penis is hypersensitive (this phenomenon is still only in the process of being scientifically documented). In a case like this, the sex therapist prescribes exercises to make the man more comfortable with erotic sensations. To begin, they focus on non-genital pleasure. Gradually, they evolve toward penetration without too much movement and then, finally, a more rhythmic penetration. By the end of the therapy, the man has learned to adjust his sexual arousal so that he can experience pleasure without triggering the ejaculation reflex," comments Mr. Goulet. He adds that premature ejaculation therapy is one of the most successful treatments (80% to 95% of cases seem to find a solution). "It is important to understand that the traditional techniques for delaying ejaculation – the stop-go technique, squeezing the end of the penis, the distraction method – are all relatively frustrating and, even though well-known around the world, not very effective."

■ SEXOANALYSIS

Sexoanalysis is a form of therapy developed approximately twenty years ago by Claude Crépault. As of yet, only a small number of sex therapists have training in this technique. Some have compared this approach to psychoanalysis because of its goal: understanding sexual disorders through analysis of the patient's erotic fantasies. In sexoanalysis, the sex therapist tries to resolve the sexual disorder by modifying the patient's problematic erotic imagination.

"According to sexoanalysis, sexual problems can spring from unresolved internal conflicts in the patient's personal history. In some cases, for example, a man's sexuality is affected by a trauma experienced in his youth: he may have been subjected to sexual abuse, a closed and strict attitude towards sex on the part of his parents, or a dominating father or mother who did not allow him to assert his masculinity. As an adult, the man may have difficulty asserting and letting himself go sexually. He may even doubt his masculinity."

Sexoanalysis (which, unlike the other approaches, is an individual process) attempts to resolve internal conflicts by working with the patient's imagination. "In essence, this approach tries to re-establish sexual health through fantasies. We invite the patient to talk about his fantasies so they can be decoded and their hidden problems corrected. This is similar to the way psychoanalysis focuses on dreams in analysis," explains Mr. Goulet.

■ HUMANISTIC-EXISTENTIAL THERAPY

This process is centred on the patient's perception of his sexual problems, rather than external appearances or the judgements of others. The patient is encouraged to get in touch with all aspects of his personality, especially his emotions. In essence, the approach teaches that we can reposition sexuality in our lives through self-knowledge. This approach is effective for all types of problems, especially diminished sex drive. It has met with particular success as a treatment for people with gender identity disorders (such as transsexuals).

"Humanistic-existential therapy can provide support for the transsexual patient going though surgery. Or, it may help the patient define his or her gender identity to the point of reconsidering surgery and deciding it is not the answer. This approach is also often used for men who doubt their masculinity and need to learn how to assert themselves for a more fully enjoyable sex life. The tools used in this process are very similar to those used in psychotherapy."

■ IS SEX THERAPY ALWAYS EFFECTIVE?

Although it is difficult to state precise success rates, we can say that the majority of couples that have undergone sex therapy have found a solution to their problem. It is, nevertheless, important to remember that the treatment can sometimes fail. The key factor in therapy is the attitude and receptivity of the patient (first and foremost) and the couple. A man who comes to see a sex therapist reluctantly – perhaps because he was given an ultimatum – and who never lets his guard down has very little chance of benefiting from the sessions. In this case, he should evaluate his true motivation before deciding what to do next. He may choose to come back at another time, or abandon therapy altogether, being conscious of the consequences to the relationship. People often refuse to see the psychological component of their problem because it seems too intimate an aspect of their personality.

"Sexuality is not only a question of the body and the emotions. It is an integral part of the personality. Therefore, if a man generally takes a lot of time to make changes in his life – for example, decides he wants to change his job, but takes three years to do it; or wants to quit smoking but can't – he will probably also have trouble modifying his unsatisfying sex life."

It can also be the case that the problem is actually what keeps the couple together. Surprising, perhaps, but it seems that it is more

VIAGRA DOES NOT NECESSARILY BUY HAPPINESS!

When sildenafil (Viagra) appeared in Canada in 1999, sex therapists thought that a drug that acted directly on erections would put an end to the practice of sex therapy. They were wrong!

Today, men who take Viagra consult sex therapists too. They know that the drug acts on them physiologically, and that it cannot help them with diminished sex drives, interpersonal relationship issues, faltering relationships, or feelings of boredom. They also know that one sex therapy treatment is cheaper than a lifetime Viagra prescription!

Men have understood that sex is not a simple question of mechanics. They know that education, values, desire, love, personal satisfaction and one's general approach to life are all parts of that complex and mysterious chemistry that is sexuality.

The clientele is also becoming younger. Frequently, patients are in their twenties or thirties. The arrival of Viagra broke down a number of barriers – in terms of general shyness and many specific taboos – and men are now more comfortable talking about what is not working in their sex lives.

common than we might think! In some relationships marked by routine, incompatibility and emotional distance, the only thing the partners have in common is their sexual problem. It has become their only possible topic of conversation. Deep down, they both know that solving the problem would change the dynamic of the relationship and likely lead to the end. If one of the two is not ready to face the problem (for example, the woman might not really want to solve the problem because it gives her a measure of control over her husband), this person may make efforts – unconsciously or not – to sabotage the therapy.

"Sometimes, sex therapy can bring about a revelation whereby the partners finally realize they no longer have any common interest in finding a solution to the problem and the relationship dissolves. Fortunately, this is very rare. Usually, the opposite is the case. Especially when it involves both partners, sex therapy can rally them around a common goal: improving their sexual satisfaction and communication," concludes Mr. Goulet.

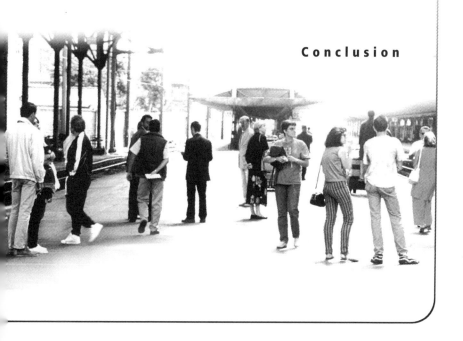

■ HOW TO CONCLUDE A BOOK ABOUT MALE SEXUAL HEALTH ?

The best way to end a book on male sexual problems is to talk about prevention, since some of the problems outlined here can be avoided or solved, at least in part, by eliminating any risk factors the man has control over.

Smokers should quit smoking. Obese men should try to lose weight by adopting healthy eating habits and doing regular physical exercise (this would also help men suffering from high cholesterol or diabetes). Men must try to lead lives that are as balanced as possible, carefully managing the time they spend at work, with their family, and enjoying recreational activities. Stabilizing these elements will take care of their physical, psychological, and personal health and will undoubtedly improve their intimate relationships and general well being.

Men should not be reluctant to take advantage of the available support by consulting a doctor or sex therapist. These health professionals have the experience and tools to help men deal with sexual dysfunction and improve their lives dramatically. Allowing shyness to interfere with finding a solution, therefore, is counter-productive, at best, and potentially dangerous, at worst.

Now you know everything there is to know about male sexuality and the various problems men can encounter. Hopefully, this book has helped men get to know themselves a little better and brought them further down the road to recovering a more satisfying sex life.